Nursing Process and Nursing Diagnosis

PATRICIA W. IYER, R.N., M.S.N.

Director of Nursing Education
Mercer Medical Center
Trenton, New Jersey

BARBARA J. TAPTICH, R.N., M.A.

Director of Education
Hamilton Hospital
Trenton, New Jersey

DONNA BERNOCCHI-LOSEY, R.N., M.A.

Instructor, University of Nevada
Las Vegas, Nevada
Formerly Assistant Director of
    Nursing—Medical-Surgical
St. Francis Medical Center
Trenton, New Jersey

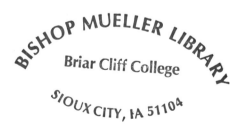

1986
W.B. SAUNDERS COMPANY
Philadelphia □ London □ Toronto □ Mexico City
Rio de Janeiro □ Sydney □ Tokyo □ Hong Kong

W. B. Saunders Company: West Washington Square
                          Philadelphia, PA   19105

Library of Congress Cataloging-in-Publication Data

Iyer, Patricia W.
  Nursing process and nursing diagnosis.

1. Nursing.   2. Diagnosis.   I. Taptich, Barbara J.   II.
   Bernocchi-Losey, Donna.   III. Title. [DNLM: 1. Nursing
   Process.   WY 100 I97n]
RT41.I94   1986   610.73   86-1062

ISBN 0-7216-1818-9

Editor: Dudley Kay
Developmental Editor: Alan Sorkowitz
Designer: Bill Donnelly
Production Manager: Bill Preston
Illustration Coordinator: Walt Verbitski
Page Layout Artist: Meg Jolly

RT
41
.I94
1986

Nursing Process and Nursing Diagnosis   ISBN   0–7216–1818–9

Last digit is the print number: 9   8   7   6   5   4   3

Dedication

To the men in our lives
who supported our ability
to complete this project:

Raj, Raj, Jr., and Nathan Iyer

Bob, Bobby, and Michael Taptich

Michael and David Losey

Preface

The nursing process is the foundation on which nursing practice is based. *Nursing Process and Nursing Diagnosis* began as a self-learning module designed to introduce the concept of the nursing diagnosis within the framework of the nursing process. We identified the need for a current, comprehensive presentation of the nursing process with an emphasis on the diagnostic phase. This text evolved from that need.

The book provides a comprehensive presentation of each of the five phases of the nursing process. The continuing emphasis on nursing diagnosis within the nursing community has been reinforced by professional standards, regulatory agencies, reimbursement systems, and the desire for a nomenclature specific to the profession. The text is particularly strong in its comprehensive discussion and utilization of the concept of the nursing diagnosis.

Nursing Process and Nursing Diagnosis is designed for nursing students and nursing practitioners wishing to learn or review nursing process theory. The material is presented in a clear, understandable fashion and provides guidelines for the development of nursing diagnoses, outcomes, and nursing orders. Exercises and case studies in a self-test format provide the learner with the opportunity to apply these concepts. Each "Test Yourself" exercise is identified by a ☑ symbol. Additionally, the symbol indicates the answer key.

The appendices include additional information that expands upon the theory contained in the body of the text.

The authors wish to thank the following reviewers, whose valuable suggestions helped to refine the content: Madelaine Lamb, Quality Assurance Coordinator, Mercer Medical Center, Trenton, New Jersey; Noranne Rowe, RN, MSN, Level I Coordinator, Mercer Medical School of Nursing, Trenton, New Jersey; Audean Duespohl, RN, MSN, MEd, Clarion State University, Venango Campus, Oil City, Pennsylvania; Ruby D. Gordon, BS, MA, PhD, Phoenix College, Phoenix, Arizona; Carol J. Bear, BSN, MEd, St. Louis Community College at Florissant Valley, St.

Louis, Missouri; Jane E. Brown, MSN, Luzerne County Community College, Nanticoke, Pennsylvania; JoAnn M. Simons, MSN, Wilkes College, Wilkes-Barre, Pennsylvania; Constance T. Welzel, RN, MA, Nassau Community College, Garden City, New York; Elizabeth Gren, RN, BS, MA, Bronson Methodist Hospital, Kalamazoo, Michigan; Mary E. Kerr, RN, BSN, MNEd, Western Pennsylvania Hospital School of Nursing, Pittsburgh, Pennsylvania; and Carol Ann Morris, MN, EdD, Northeastern Oklahoma A&M College, Miami, Oklahoma. Additionally, we appreciate the skill and patience of Dorothy Battershell, who typed the manuscript. A special thanks is directed to Dudley Kay, Publisher, WB Saunders, who also recognized the need for this text and encouraged us in our efforts.

Contents

1

The Nursing Process

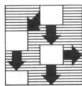

INTRODUCTION

Early nursing practice encompassed many roles. The nurse focused on comfort measures and maintaining a sanitary environment. In addition, the roles of pharmacist, dietician, physical therapist, and social worker were part of nursing practice. The nurse as a health care provider met the total needs of the client. Since that time, there have been a number of factors that have altered the dimensions of nursing practice. These include social, scientific/technological, educational, economic, and political changes. During the evolutionary process, the common thread that has remained is the nurse's focus on the total needs of the client. However, the previously identified factors have also changed the complexion of health care in general. A variety of disciplines have evolved to assist in meeting client needs—physical therapy, social services, dietetics. The role of the nurse in the delivery of these ancillary services has shifted from provider to coordinator. This allows the nurse to concentrate on the body of knowledge unique to nursing in the resolution of client problems. The method by which this is accomplished is the "nursing process." It may be helpful to explore some definitions of nursing prior to examining the nursing process in detail.

DEFINITIONS OF NURSING

The profession of nursing has been defined by nursing leaders, by professional organizations, and according to functions.

Nursing Leaders

The earliest definition of nursing was provided by Florence Nightingale in 1859. Nightingale's *Notes on Nursing—What It Is, What It Is Not*—defined nursing as having "charge of the personal health of somebody . . . and what nursing has to do . . . is to put the patient in the best condition for nature to act upon him." The nature of nursing is complex, and efforts to define it have continued. A frequently quoted definition, used internationally, was formulated by Virginia Henderson (1961). She viewed nursing as assisting "the individual, sick or well, in the performance of those activities contributing to health or its recovery (or to peaceful death) that he would perform unaided if he had the necessary strength, will or knowledge."

Claire Fagin (1978) suggests that "nursing is defined as including the promotion and maintenance of health, prevention of illness, care of persons during acute phases of illness, and rehabilitation and restoration of health." Orlando (1961) viewed nursing as providing "the help the patient may require for his needs to be met, that is, for his physical and mental comfort to be assured as far as possible."

Martha Rogers (1970) describes nursing as both an art and a science. She further identifies the existence of a unique knowledge base "growing out of scientific research and logical analysis and capable of being translated into nursing practice."

These definitions are just a sample of the many descriptions of nursing. It could be summarized that nursing is both a science and an art. Nursing has its own body of knowledge based on scientific theory and focuses on the health and well-being of the client. Nursing is concerned with the psychological, spiritual, social, and physical aspects of the person, rather than only the client's diagnosed medical condition. In other words, the focus is on the responses of the total person interacting with the environment. These responses may be influenced by past experiences, the physical environment, the social situation, and family dynamics. Nursing is an art that involves caring for the client during times of illness and assisting the client to achieve maximum health potential throughout the life cycle. Nursing strives to adapt to the needs of people through personal interaction with individuals, families, and communities in a variety of settings—home, work, clinics, and hospitals.

Professional Organizations

The mission of defining nursing has been undertaken by others besides nurse leaders. In 1979, the American Nurses' Association, the professional organization for nursing in the United States, defined nursing and established the scope of nursing practice. The end result of the ANA's efforts was the publication of Nursing: A Social Policy Statement (1980). The definition of nursing presented in this document reflected the historical evolution of the profession and its theoretical base: "Nursing is the diagnosis and treatment of human responses to actual or potential health problems."

Human Responses

Human responses are the phenomena of concern to nurses. The nurse focuses on two types of responses: "(1) reactions of individuals and groups to actual health problems (health-restoring responses), such as the impact of illness—effects upon the self and family, and self-care needs; and (2) concerns of individuals and groups about potential health problems (health supporting responses), such as monitoring and teaching in populations or communities at risk in which educative needs for information, skill development, health-oriented attitudes and related behavioral changes arise" (ANA, 1980). More simply, this means that the scope of nursing practice includes the tasks of assessing, diagnosing and treating, and evaluating the responses observed in both sick and well persons. Nursing interventions can be directed to the management of the response to an actual problem, such as an illness or disease, or the prevention of a health problem in a client at risk. In short, the nurse deals with the client's response to the health problem. The nurse is concerned with the effect of the disease or health problem on the client's life. These human responses are dynamic in nature and change as the client and/or family progresses along the continuum between health and illness. The client usually has one or more human responses to an acute illness or long-term disease. The human responses are diverse and vary in nature because each client is a unique individual, and the response to the health problem or potential health problem will be a reflection of the individual's interaction with the environment. Consider the following situation.

Example. Mr. Vegas is a 52 year old cross-country truck driver. While driving his truck 1000 miles from home, he began to develop some tightness in his chest. At first, he passed it off as indigestion. When the discomfort failed to dissipate, he drove to the nearest hospital. Mr. Vegas was admitted to the intensive care unit with severe chest pain. He was restless and withdrawn. Later, he said that this was his first time in the hospital and he was afraid he might die. He asked the nurse to call his wife to ask her to come as quickly as possible. Fortunately, Mr. Vegas had an uncomplicated heart attack. After a few days, he was transferred to another floor. While the nurse was transferring him, Mr. Vegas expressed his concern over the fact that he was going to a new unit. Once on the unit, the physician informed him that it would be in his best interest to change his lifestyle and perhaps retire from truck driving. Mr. Vegas stated that this was impossible for he had no other way to support his wife and four children.

This example demonstrates some of the human responses Mr. Vegas had to the health problem of a heart attack. During his hospitalization, the medical diagnosis remained the same from the time of admission to discharge. However, the human responses were multiple in nature and varied based on his progress along the health care continuum. Upon admission, the responses exhibited were those of pain, fear of death, and loneliness. As his health status improved, he exhibited anxiety about his transfer and had difficulty in accepting the major change in lifestyle suggested by the physician. The nurse's role was to identify the responses of pain, fear, loneliness, and anxiety and to assist the client in managing them. These are the types of human responses that are within the realm of nursing practice.

Table 1–1 is an illustration of some of the human responses that are the focus for nursing intervention.

TABLE 1–1 □ **HUMAN RESPONSES**

1. Self-care limitations
2. Impaired functioning in areas such as rest, sleep, ventilation, circulation, activity, nutrition, elimination, skin, sexuality
3. Pain and discomfort
4. Emotional problems related to illness and treatment, life-threatening events, or daily experiences, such as anxiety, loss, loneliness, and grief
5. Distortion of symbolic functions, reflected in interpersonal and intellectual processes, such as hallucinations
6. Deficiencies in decision-making and ability to make personal choices
7. Self-image changes required by health status
8. Dysfunctional perceptual orientation to health
9. Strains related to life processes, such as birth, growth and development, and death
10. Problematic affiliative relationships

Reprinted with permission of the American Nurses' Association. From Nursing: A Social Policy Statement. Kansas City, MO: American Nurses' Association, 1980.

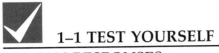

1–1 TEST YOURSELF

HUMAN RESPONSES

After reading the situation below, identify four human responses to actual or potential health problems.

Mrs. Hart was a 32 year old white female admitted to the acute care facility with a lump in her right breast. Mrs. Hart informed the nurse that her husband had noticed the lump in her breast approximately six months ago. She had put off going to the doctor because she was afraid that it might be cancer. She explained that she had a two year old child at home and was hoping to become pregnant in the near future, but now that the lump had been discovered, her own future was in doubt. She had delayed childbirth because of her career as an accountant. During the conversation she became teary-eyed. After questioning her, the nurse determined that she had never had surgery before and was anxious about receiving anesthesia. Her only admission to a hospital had been for the delivery of her child utilizing natural childbirth techniques.

Mrs. Hart went to the operating room the next day and underwent a right modified mastectomy. On her first day following surgery, she experienced much pain, and because of the nature of the surgery her ability to move her right arm was impaired. This was disturbing to her since she was right-handed. She was not accustomed to being so dependent. On the fourth day after surgery, the physician informed Mrs. Hart that because the disease had spread to two lymph nodes she would require chemotherapy, radiation therapy, or both. After the physician left, Mrs. Hart broke down and started to cry. She told the nurse that she was afraid she would never be able to have another child or see her little girl grow up. She also refused to look at her incision when the dressing was changed and expressed that she was scarred for life and would never be attractive to her husband again.

Human Responses

1.

2.

3.

4.

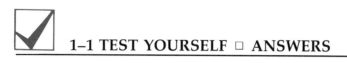

1–1 TEST YOURSELF □ ANSWERS

1. Self-care limitations
2. Pain
3. Fear of surgery/anesthesia
4. Fear of death
5. Change in self-image
6. Change in relationship with husband
7. Impaired sexuality
8. Grief

Nursing Functions

Nursing has also been defined in terms of functions or roles. In nursing practice, the roles can be divided into three areas: independent, interdependent, and dependent functions.

Independent Functions

Independent functions are those activities that are considered to be within nursing's scope of diagnosis and treatment. These actions do not require a physician's order. Some examples include:

1. Assessment of the client/family through health history and physical examination to ascertain health status;

2. Diagnosis of responses requiring nursing interventions;

3. Identification of nursing actions that are likely to maintain or restore health;

4. Implementation of measures designed to motivate, guide, support, counsel, or teach the client/family;

5. Referral to other members of the health care team when indicated and allowed by individual state nurse practice acts;

6. Evaluation of the client's response to nursing and medical interventions;

7. Participation with consumers or other health care providers in the improvement of health care systems.

Interdependent Functions

The interdependent functions of the nurse are those that are carried out in conjunction with other health team members. For example, in the case of a pregnant diabetic in a high-risk clinic, the nurse and dietician collaborate to develop a plan for meeting the nutritional needs of the expectant mother and developing fetus. The dietician contributes in meal planning and teaching, while the nurse reinforces the teaching and monitors the client's ability to incorporate the diet into daily food selection. Another example might be seen in the physician's office. The physician diagnoses the medical problem of hypertension and orders medications and dietary modifications in an elderly client. In response to the physician's findings, the office nurse assesses the client's reaction to the diagnosis and initiates teaching about disease, drugs, and diet. These are examples of the interdependent functions of the nurse.

Dependent Functions

The dependent functions of the nurse are the activities performed based on the physician's orders. These include the administration of medications or specific treatments. For example, in a hospital pediatric unit, the nurse recognizes a temperature elevation in a child with gastroenteritis. In this setting, it is not within the scope of nursing practice to order antipyretics and intravenous fluids. However, when these treatment modalities are ordered by the physician, it is the nurse's responsibility to administer the medication and initiate intravenous therapy. These are the dependent functions of the nurse.

It is important to note that each state has legally defined the practice of nursing in its Nursing Practice Act. Once licensed, the nurse is responsible and accountable for practicing nursing within the state's legal definition. For example, the practice of nursing, as described by the New Jersey State Board of Nursing in its Nurse Practice Act (1975), is clearly defined in terms of its independent, interdependent, and dependent roles. It states:

Independent and Interdependent Functions	"The practice of nursing as a registered professional nurse is defined as diagnosing and treating human responses to actual or potential physical and emotional health problems through such services as casefinding, health teaching, health counseling, and provision of care supportive to or restorative of life and well being. . .
Dependent Functions	. . . and executing medical regimen as prescribed by a licensed or otherwise legally authorized physician or dentist."

Case Study

Mr. Rubin Paul, age 64, was five days post-op after bowel surgery for cancer. While caring for Mr. Paul, the nurse noted he was withdrawn and noncommunicative. The client's wife verbalized her concern about this dramatic change in her husband's behavior. The nurse discussed this information with the surgeon, and they reached a mutual agreement that a psychiatric evaluation would benefit Mr. Paul. The client and his wife agreed, and the physician ordered a psychiatric consultation. The nurse notified the consultant and shared information pertinent to Mr. Paul's physical and psychological status. The psychiatrist evaluated the client, confirmed the diagnosis of post-op depression, and ordered medications. The nurse incorporated the administration of this medication along with the use of therapeutic communication into the client's plan of care. In addition, the nurse monitored Mr. Paul's response to both of these modalities.

The following lists identify the independent, interdependent, and dependent functions that the nurse performed in this case study.

Independent	Interdependent	Dependent
1. Assessment of psychological status (withdrawn and noncommunicative)	1. Discussion with surgeon regarding psychiatric evaluation	1. Administration of medication
2. Therapeutic communication	2. Communication with psychiatrist about physical and psychological status	
3. Evaluation for response to medication and therapeutic communication		

In conclusion, the practice of nursing has been defined by nursing leaders, by professional organizations, and according to function to include independent, interdependent, and dependent functions. This definition will continue to evolve in response to nursing research and theory building as well as to the increasing complexity of health care. However, meeting the total needs of the client will continue to be the focus of nursing practice.

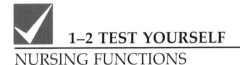

1–2 TEST YOURSELF

NURSING FUNCTIONS

The following situation will give you a chance to practice identifying the independent, interdependent, and dependent functions of the registered nurse. After reading the scenario, identify three independent, one interdependent, and three dependent functions of the nurse.

Mr. Ease was an 84 year old white male admitted to your unit at 6 AM. The night charge nurse reported that Mr. Ease had a history of urinary incontinence at home. His skin was intact, but she noted a reddened area approximately two inches in diameter at the base of his spine. He had limited range of motion in all his extremities and was unable to reposition himself in bed.

On first rounds, the nurse found Mrs. Ease, his 80 year old wife, outside the room crying. She stated that she was worried about what was going to happen to her husband since they had no children and she could no longer care for him.

Based on the physician's physical exam and information obtained from the nurse, some of the physician's orders included: intravenous therapy, vital signs every four hours, two acetaminophen (Tylenol) by mouth every four hours for a temperature elevation above 102°F, insertion of Foley urinary catheter, and consultation with physical therapy.

During the course of the day, Mr. Ease's temperature was elevated to 103°F (rectally). The nurse administered the Tylenol and decided to monitor the client's vital signs every hour for the next three hours. The nurse inserted the Foley catheter, placed a four inch foam mattress on the bed, and established a turning schedule. Intravenous therapy and intake and output recording were initiated. The physical therapy department was notified, and a social service referral was made by the nurse. After the physical therapy consultation, a regimen for range of motion exercises was established. This included bedside physical therapy twice a day on the day shift by the therapist and specific active and passive exercises on the evening shift by the nursing staff.

Independent	**Interdependent**	**Dependent**
1.	1.	1.
2.		2.
3.		3.

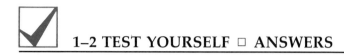

1–2 TEST YOURSELF □ ANSWERS

Independent	Interdependent	Dependent
1. Increasing frequency of vital sign measurements	1. Performing active and passive range of motion exercises as suggested by physical therapy	1. Measuring and recording vital signs every four hours
2. Initiating intake and output recording		2. Administering medications
3. Assessing need for skin protection measures		3. Initiating intravenous therapy
4. Establishing a turning schedule and applying a foam mattress		4. Inserting Foley catheter
5. Social service referral		

THE NURSING PROCESS

The science of nursing is based on a broad theoretical framework. The nursing process is the method by which this framework is applied to the practice of nursing. It is a deliberative problem-solving approach that requires cognitive, technical, and interpersonal skills and is directed to meeting the needs of the client/family system (Smith and Germain, 1975). The nursing process consists of five sequential and interrelated phases—assessment, diagnosis, planning, implementation, and evaluation. These phases integrate the intellectual functions of problem-solving in an effort to define nursing actions.

History

The nursing process has evolved into a five step process consistent with the developing nature of the profession. It was first described as a distinct process by Hall (1955). Johnson (1959), Orlando (1961), and Wiedenbach (1963) each developed a different three step process that contained rudimentary elements of the five step process. In 1967, Yura and Walsh authored the first text that described a four phase process—assessment, planning, implementation, and evaluation. In the mid-1970s, Bloch (1974), Roy (1975), Mundinger and Jauron (1975), and Aspinall (1976) added the diagnostic phase, resulting in a five step process.

Since that time, the nursing process has been legitimized as the framework of nursing practice. The American Nurses' Association used the nursing process as a guideline in developing the Standards of Nursing Practice. The nursing process has been incorporated into the conceptual framework of most nursing curriculums. It has also been included in the definition of nursing in the majority of nurse practice acts. More recently, the state board examinations were revised to test the ability of the aspiring registered nurse to utilize the steps of the nursing process.

Definition

The nursing process can be defined in terms of three major dimensions: purpose, organization, and properties.

Purpose

The major purpose of the nursing process is to provide a framework within which the individualized needs of the client, family, and community can be met. Yura and Walsh (1983) state that "the nursing process is the designated series of actions intended to fulfill the purpose of nursing—to maintain the client's optimal wellness—and, if this state changes, to provide the amount and quality of nursing care his situation demands to direct him back to wellness. If wellness cannot be achieved, the nursing process should contribute to the client's quality of life maximizing his resources to achieve the highest quality of living possible for as long a time as possible."

The nursing process involves an interactional relationship between the client and the nurse, with the client as the focus. The nurse validates observations with the client, and together they utilize the process. This assists the client to deal with actual or potential changes in health and results in individualized care.

Organization

As noted above, the nursing process is organized into five identifiable phases—assessment, diagnosis, planning, implementation, and evaluation. Each can be further described as follows.

Assessment. Assessment is the first phase of the nursing process. Its activities are focused on gathering information regarding the client, the client/family system, or the community for the purpose of identifying the client's needs, problems, concerns, or human responses. Data are collected in a systematic fashion, utilizing the interview or nursing history, physical examination, laboratory results, and other sources.

Diagnosis. During this phase, the data collected during assessment are critically analyzed and interpreted. Conclusions are drawn regarding the client's needs, problems, concerns, and human responses. The nursing diagnoses are identified and provide a central focus for the remainder of the phases. Based on the nursing diagnoses, the plan of care is designed, implemented, and evaluated. The nursing diagnoses supply an efficient method of communicating the client's problems.

Planning. In the planning phase, strategies are developed to prevent, minimize, or correct the problems identified in the nursing diagnosis. The planning phase consists of several steps:

    1. Establishing priorities for the problems diagnosed

    2. Setting outcomes with the client to correct, minimize, or prevent the problems

    3. Writing nursing orders that will lead to the achievement of the proposed outcomes

    4. Recording nursing diagnoses, outcomes, and nursing actions in an organized fashion on the care plan.

Implementation. Implementation is the initiation and completion of the actions necessary to achieve the outcomes defined in the planning stage. It involves communication of the plan to all those participating in the client's care. The interventions can be carried out by members of the health team, the client, or the client's family. The plan of care is used as a guide. The nurse continues to collect data regarding the client's condition and interaction with the environment. Implementation also includes recording the patient's care on the proper documents. This documentation verifies that the plan of care has been carried out and can be used as a tool to evaluate the plan's effectiveness.

Evaluation. The last phase of the nursing process is evaluation. It is an ongoing process that determines the extent to which the goals of care have been achieved. The nurse assesses the progress of the client, institutes corrective measures if required, and revises the nursing care plan.

    This discussion has separated the nursing process into five distinct phases. In actual practice, it is impossible to separate the phases because they are interrelated and interdependent.

Properties

The nursing process has six properties. It is purposeful, systematic, dynamic, interactive, flexible, and theoretically based. The nursing process can be described as purposeful because it is goal directed. The nurse utilizes the phases of the process to provide quality client-centered care. The process is systematic because it involves the use of an organized approach to achieve its purpose. This deliberate method promotes the quality of nursing and avoids the problems associated with intuition or traditional care delivery.

The nursing process is dynamic because it involves continuous change. It is an ongoing process focused on the changing responses of the client that are identified throughout the nurse-client relationship. The interactive nature of the nursing process is based on the reciprocal relationships that occur between the nurse and the client, family, and other health professionals. This component ensures the individualization of client care.

The flexibility of the process may be demonstrated in two contexts: (1) it can be adapted to nursing practice in any setting or area of specialization dealing with individuals, groups, or communities; (2) its phases may be used sequentially and concurrently. The nursing process is most frequently utilized in sequence; however, the nurse may utilize more than one step at a time. For example, while implementing the plan, the nurse may assess the client to evaluate the plan's effectiveness.

Finally, the nursing process is theoretically based. The process is devised from a broad base of knowledge, including the sciences and humanities, and can be applied to any of the theoretical models of nursing.

IMPLICATIONS OF THE NURSING PROCESS

The use of the nursing process in practice has implications for the profession of nursing, the client, and the individual nurse.

Implications for the Profession

Professionally, the nursing process concretely demonstrates the scope of nursing practice. Through the five phases, nursing continues to define its role to the consumer and other health care professionals. This clearly points out that the realm of nursing is more than just implementing the plan of care as prescribed by the physician.

TABLE 1–2 □ GENERIC STANDARDS OF PRACTICE

I. The collection of data about the health status of the client/patient is systematic and continuous. The data are accessible, communicated, and recorded.
II. The nursing diagnosis is derived from health status data.
III. The plan of nursing care includes goals derived from the nursing diagnosis.
IV. The plan of nursing care includes priorities and prescribed nursing approaches or measures to achieve goals derived from the nursing diagnosis.
V. Nursing actions provide for patient participation in health promotions, maintenance, and restoration.
VI. Nursing actions assist the patient to maximize his health capabilities.
VII. The patient's progress or lack of progress toward goal achievement is determined by the patient and the nurse.
VIII. The patient's progress or lack of progress toward goal achievement directs reassessment, recording of priorities, new goal setting, and revision of the plan of nursing care.

Reprinted with permission of the American Nurses' Association. From Standards of Nursing Practice. Kansas City, MO: American Nurses' Association, 1973.

In addition, the nursing process has been incorporated into standards of practice. These standards were adopted and published by the American Nurses' Association (Table 1–2). Nurses are held accountable for practicing according to these standards regardless of the setting or their area of specialization. Additional standards have been formulated by the ANA Divisions of Practice (Maternal-Child Health, Gerontology, Psychiatric Mental Health, Community Health, etc.).

Implications for the Client

The use of the nursing process benefits the client and family. It encourages them to participate actively in care by involving them in all five phases of the process. The client provides assessment data, validates the nursing diagnosis, confirms outcomes and interventions, assists with implementation, and provides feedback for evaluation. In addition, the written plan promotes continuity of care, which results in a safe, therapeutic environment. The absence of this continuity may cause problems similar to those described in the following situation.

Example. Ms. Dean was a nursing supervisor of a Medical-Surgical Unit. On rounds, she encountered Mrs. Martin, the wife of one of the clients, who stated that she had some complaints concerning the care of her husband. She explained that her husband developed an infection of his incision following bowel surgery. The doctor told her the dressing had to be changed and the wound irrigated three times daily. She indicated that this procedure was being done but that each nurse did it differently.

Some even asked her or her husband how to do the procedure. "How come the nurses don't all do it the same? Who is doing it right? Shouldn't it be written somewhere? How will my husband ever get better?"

This situation demonstrates that when nursing care is uncoordinated, the family loses confidence in the staff's ability to meet the client's needs. An anxiety-producing environment is created rather than a therapeutic one.

The use of a systematic method of providing nursing care also improves the quality of that care. The absence of this type of approach can lead to error, omissions, and duplications in care.

Example. Mrs. Azzari, a 30 year old teacher, delivered her second child a week ago. Usually the public health nurse's first visit includes teaching about growth and development and contraception. However, the nurse's assessment of this client's learning needs revealed adequate understanding in both of these areas. Therefore teaching focused on providing information about infant nutrition—a topic of concern to the client.

The use of the nursing process in this situation ensured a thorough assessment of the client's learning needs and involved her in planning approaches to meet them. Failure to do so might have resulted in a frustrating experience for the client, which also could compromise the quality of care delivered.

Individualized care is also promoted by the use of the nursing process. For example, the priorities of care for a client with pneumonia frequently focus on temperature monitoring, hydration, and antibiotic therapy. When Bonnie Zuckerman was admitted for pneumonia, her three preschool children were left with a 15 year old baby sitter. The physician's plan of care included temperature control, intravenous therapy, and antibiotics. In the assessment phase, the nurse identified Bonnie's concern about her children. Because of her child care problem, Bonnie felt she had no choice but to leave the hospital against medical advice. The nurse initiated a social service consultation that resolved Bonnie's dilemma. This allowed Bonnie to remain in the hospital and to participate in those measures designed to restore her health. By looking at Bonnie's special needs, the nurse was able to provide quality individualized care.

The need for individualized care is further supported by the licensing or accrediting agencies. For instance, the Joint Commission on Accreditation of Hospitals is an independent agency that reviews health care facilities to evaluate the quality of care provided. The Joint Commission Standard IV for Nursing (1985) states "Individualized goal directed nursing care shall be provided to patients through the use of the nursing process." Accreditation by this agency ensures the consumer that quality health care is provided by the facility.

Implications for the Nurse

The nursing process increases job satisfaction and enhances professional growth. The development of meaningful nurse-client relationships is facilitated by the nursing process. The rewards obtained from nursing practice are frequently derived from the nurse's ability to assist the client to meet identified needs. The genuine "thank you," regardless of the manner in which it is expressed by clients and their families, often outweighs any other type of recognition.

The nursing process encourages innovation and creativity in solving nursing care problems. This prevents the boredom that could result from a repetitive, task-oriented approach.

Example. Consider the case of Karen and Glenn Stanton, who were seen in the Emergency Department with multiple injuries after a car accident. The nurse determined that Mr. and Mrs. Stanton were extremely apprehensive about being separated from each other. The traditional approach of admitting them to separate rooms would add additional stress and interfere with their recuperation. Therefore, the nurse requested that the admitting department place the couple in the same room. Upon discharge, the couple expressed their appreciation.

This creative intervention hastened their recovery and provided the nurse with a sense of accomplishment.

Job satisfaction may also be increased through the use of the care plan developed from the nursing process. Well-written care plans save time and energy and prevent the frustration that is generated by trial and error nursing. Consider this situation.

Example. Mr. Lodge was a 300 lb man who had a right total hip replacement three days ago. Today the nurse caring for him must get him out of bed. The nurse giving change of shift report stated that yesterday was his first time out of bed. The nurse was concerned about how she was going to accomplish this task. She knew that Mr. Lodge was overweight, could not bear weight on the right leg, and was at risk for dislocating his hip. She was familiar with several recommended procedures for getting the client out of bed safely; however, the chart and care plan gave no indication of which method was successfully used on the previous day. Mr. Lodge was unable to describe the method used, and the nurses who assisted him were not available. The nurse finally selected a strategy, chose a chair, and estimated the amount of assistance she would need to move Mr. Lodge.

This situation illustrates how the nursing care plan can save time and decrease frustration. In this instance, if the care plan had specified directions on how to get Mr. Lodge out of bed, the nurse would not have experienced frustration and anger. She would have been able to get Mr. Lodge out of bed more efficiently. As demonstrated here, coordinating a client's nursing care through the use of a care plan greatly increases the chances of achieving the desired outcome.

The nursing process enhances professional growth. The application of the nursing process encourages the development of cognitive, technical, and interpersonal skills. The nurse accumulates additional knowledge through interaction with colleagues, clients, and other health care providers. The nursing process increases the potential for accurate identification of the client's response and implementation of appropriate actions. Nursing audits are used to examine the care provided, compare it to predetermined standards, and identify strengths and weaknesses. This assures quality care and suggests areas requiring additional education or development. Interaction with a variety of clients and other health care professionals encourages refinement of the nurse's verbal and nonverbal communication skills. The effectiveness of the nurse in daily practice is therefore enhanced.

SUMMARY

The dimensions of nursing practice have evolved in response to the scientific/technological, educational, economic, and political changes in society. The practice of nursing has been defined by nursing leaders, by professional organizations, and by regulatory agencies.

The nursing process is the method by which the theoretical frameworks of nursing are applied to actual practice. It can be defined in terms of three major dimensions: purpose, organization, and properties. The nursing process provides the framework to meet the individualized needs of the client, family, and community. It can be organized into five phases—assessment, diagnosis, planning, implementation, and evaluation. It has been characterized as purposeful, systematic, dynamic, interactive, flexible, and theoretically based.

The use of the nursing process has implications for the profession of nursing, the client, and the individual nurse. Professionally the nursing process defines the scope of nursing practice and identifies standards of nursing care. The client benefits by the use of the nursing process, since it ensures quality care while encouraging the client to participate in care. Finally, the benefits for the individual nurse are increased job satisfaction and enhancement of professional growth.

References

American Nurses' Association: Standards of Nursing Practice. Kansas City, MO: American Nurses' Association, 1973.

American Nurses' Association: Nursing: A Social Policy Statement. Kansas City, MO: American Nurses' Association, 1980.

Aspinall, MJ: Nursing diagnosis—the weak link. Nursing Outlook 24:433–437, 1976.

Bloch D: Some crucial terms in nursing—what do they really mean? Nursing Outlook 22:689–694, 1974.

Fagin C: Primary care as an academic discipline. Nursing Outlook 26:750–753, 1978.

Hall LE: Quality of nursing care. Public Health News, June 1955.

Henderson V: Basic principles of nursing care. London: International Council of Nurses, 1961.

Johnson D: A philosophy for nursing diagnosis. Nursing Outlook 7(4):198–200, 1959.

Joint Commission on Accredition of Hospitals: AMH/85: Accreditation Manual For Hospitals. Chicago: Joint Commission on Accreditation of Hospitals, 1985.

Mundinger M and Jauron G: Developing a nursing diagnosis. Nursing Outlook 23:94–98, 1975.

Nightingale F: Notes on Nursing. What It Is, What It Is Not. New York: Dover Publications, 1969. (Originally published, 1859).

Orlando I: The Dynamic Nurse-Patient Relationship. New York: GP Putnam's Sons, 1961.

Rogers ME: Nursing Science: Introduction to the Theoretical Basis of Nursing. Philadelphia: FA Davis, 1970.

Roy C: The impact of nursing diagnosis. American Operating Room Nurses Journal 21(5):1023–1030, 1975.

Schlotfeldt R: The professional doctorate: rationale and characteristics. Nursing Outlook 26:(5):302–311, 1978.

Smith DW and Germain CP: Care of the Adult Patient. 4th ed. Philadelphia: JP Lippincott, 1975.

State of New Jersey Nursing Practice Act. Newark: New Jersey State Board of Nursing, 1975.

Wiedenbach E: The helping art of nursing. American Journal of Nursing 63(11):54–57, 1963.

Yura H and Walsh M: The Nursing Process: Assessing, Planning, Implementing, Evaluation. 1st ed. New York: Appleton-Century-Crofts, 1967.

Yura H and Walsh MB: The Nursing Process: Assessing, Planning, Implementing, Evaluation. 4th ed. New York: Appleton-Century-Crofts, 1983.

Bibliography

Beland I and Passos JY: Clinical Nursing: Pathophysiological and Psychosocial Approaches. 4th ed. New York: Macmillan Publishing Co., Inc., 1981.

Carlson JH, Craft C, and McGuire AD (eds): Nursing Diagnosis. Philadelphia: WB Saunders Company, 1982.

Griffith J and Christensen P: Nursing Process: Application of Theories, Framework and Models. St. Louis: CV Mosby, 1982.

Kelly LY: Dimensions of Professional Nursing. 4th ed. New York: Macmillan Publishing Co., Inc., 1981.

LaMonica EL: The Nursing Process: A Humanistic Approach. Menlo Park: Addison-Wesley Publishing Co., 1979.

2

Assessment

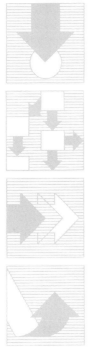

Assessment is the first step of the nursing process and can be described as the organized and systematic process of collecting data from a variety of sources to evaluate the health status of a client. The importance of this phase of the nursing process has been addressed specifically in the Standards of Nursing Practice of the American Nurses' Association. The first standard defines the need for the systematic collection of data that are accessible to health care providers (ANA, 1973). The fact that the assessment standard is the first of the eight standards is significant in reinforcing its importance as the key to the remaining steps of the process.

The assessment phase provides a solid foundation that promotes the delivery of quality individualized care. Accurate, complete assessment is necessary to facilitate the diagnosis and treatment of human responses—the scope of nursing practice as defined by the ANA (1980). Assessment forms the basis for the identification of nursing diagnoses, development of outcomes, implementation of nursing orders, and evaluation of nursing interventions.

The initial assessment enables the nurse to accumulate comprehensive data about health problems. It also helps to identify the specific factors that contribute to the existence of these problems in an individual client. This encourages the nurse and client to develop outcomes. It also facilitates the implementation of nursing

19

interventions designed to achieve the outcomes. Subsequent assessments validate the existence of previously identified concerns and document the client's progress toward the outcomes. These data also determine whether the nurse should change, expand, or discontinue nursing interventions. Since assessment is a continuous process, subsequent data also allow the nurse to identify additional problems that may have developed as a result of hospitalization, the disease process, or treatment modalities. This is accomplished through a process that compares current information to previously acquired baseline data.

PREREQUISITES

Beliefs

The nurse's beliefs include philosophies about nursing, health, the client as an individual and as a health care consumer, and the interactions between these factors. These become part of the theoretical framework upon which the nurse's practice is based. This framework is reflected not only in the assessment phase but also throughout the remaining components of the nursing process.

Example. Steven Bodine, age 25, is admitted to the hospital with a medical diagnosis of metastatic cancer of the lung. His primary site, testicular cancer, was diagnosed three years ago, and he has completed an extended series of both radiation and drug therapies. Steven and his wife have reached a mutual decision that his disease process and the need for continuing therapy have severely affected the quality of his life. Therefore, he has chosen to discontinue all therapy. This decision is supported by his physician.

The nurse believes that Steven has the right to make an informed decision and to control the manner in which he spends the remainder of his life. His nurse also believes that a nurse's goal as a client advocate is to assist him to accomplish these goals. The assessment phase identifies that Steven would like to be made comfortable and to die at home with the support of his family. The nurse's interventions would therefore focus on the implementation of a pain management regime, patient/family teaching, and referral to a hospice program.

Knowledge

The process of assessment demands that the nurse possess an extensive body of knowledge from a variety of disciplines. This knowledge base includes both physical and behavioral sciences. The nurse is expected to master basic concepts of anatomy, physiology, chemistry, nutrition, microbiology, psychology, and sociology. The components of this scientific base allow the nurse to make the initial assessment of the client's physiological and psychological state. Such a body of knowledge also forms the basis for recognition of change during subsequent assessments. This facilitates the identification of contributing factors, both positive and negative, that determine the client's position on the health/illness continuum.

The nurse's knowledge base must also include the fundamentals of problem-solving, analysis, and decision-making. The nurse must be able to analyze assessment data, recognize significant relationships among data, develop valid conclusions, and subsequently make sound nursing judgments that contribute to the client's progress.

Example. John Thomas is an obese 42 year old salesman who is admitted to the hospital for a cholecystectomy. On the third post-op day, Mr. Thomas calls the nurse and indicates that he feels as though his "stitches are popping." The nurse notes that he is pale and diaphoretic, and further observation reveals four open sutures in the incisional area. A loop of bowel is protruding through the lower end of the opening. In addition, the client is hypotensive, with a blood pressure of 100/68.

Based on this assessment, the nurse instructs the client not to eat or drink, places a sterile saline-soaked dressing over his abdomen, and contacts Mr. Thomas's surgeon. The nurse's knowledge base is used to anticipate the need for further surgery. Her problem-solving skills resulted in prompt nursing actions that prevented more serious complications.

Skills

A variety of skills are necessary for the nurse to complete an effective assessment. These skills are related to the knowledge base and may be both technical and interpersonal in nature.

Technical skills associated with the assessment phase involve specific techniques and procedures that allow the nurse to collect the data. Some are associated with the use of equipment such as stethoscopes, sphygmomanometers, and thermometers for the measurement of vital signs. Other technical skills involve the performance of procedures such as palpation of pulses or auscultation of heart, lung, or bowel sounds. Both types of technical skills are required for accurate, complete assessment.

Interpersonal skills are important during all phases of the nursing process but are particularly critical to successful assessment. Since this is a communicative, interactive process, the nurse must have highly developed communication skills. These facilitate the development of positive relationships between the nurse and client or family. These relationships allow the nurse to

☐ Determine what the client/family sees as priorities
☐ Identify additional nursing concerns
☐ Create a therapeutic environment in which mutual outcomes may be accomplished.

The therapeutic environment begins to develop during assessment and requires the nurse to possess verbal and nonverbal communication abilities. Certainly, the nurse must be able to share information with the client by choosing language that accurately conveys the desired message at a level appropriate for the client. In addition, the nurse must have highly developed listening skills, which contribute to the therapeutic environment by allowing the client to feel comfortable expressing thoughts, feelings, and concerns. The nonverbal component of communication is of particular importance in the assessment process and the development of nurse-client relationships.

Creativity, common sense, and flexibility are additional interpersonal skills required when assessing the client/family. The nurse is frequently required to be creative in developing strategies to facilitate assessment. This is particularly important when clients are very young or frightened or have communication barriers.

Example. Cindy is a three year old who was brought to the university clinic by her mother. She is complaining of abdominal pain and is obviously frightened. Cindy screams when the nurse attempts to examine her abdomen. The nurse asks Cindy to show where it hurts on her doll or on mommy. This creative approach allows the nurse to obtain information in a manner that is much less threatening to Cindy.

Common sense dictates that detailed nursing histories should be postponed on clients who are experiencing acute anxiety, pain, or dyspnea. This creates an environment of sensitivity and caring, which may also be evidenced by the nurse's flexibility in responding to client requests.

Example. Nora York is a 61 year old woman admitted for elective knee joint replacement. The nurse greets her, makes her comfortable, and begins the nursing history. Mrs. York indicates that she would prefer that her daughter, a nurse, be with her during the interview and that she expects her within an hour.

In this situation, the nurse demonstrates flexibility in selecting the timing of the health history. This sensitivity puts Mrs. York at ease and strengthens the nurse's relationship with this client.

The assessment phase is affected by the nurse's beliefs, knowledge, and skills. The nurse's philosophies form the foundation for nurse-client interactions. Knowledge and skills are the tools that enable the nurse to accumulate data, determine their significance, and develop interventions that reflect quality individualized nursing care.

COMPONENTS OF THE ASSESSMENT PHASE

The assessment process consists of two basic components—data collection and documentation.

Data Collection

In the context of the nursing assessment, data might be defined as specific information obtained about a client. The nurse systematically accumulates the information required to diagnose the client's unhealthful responses and to identify contributing factors. This data base subsequently forms the foundation for the remaining phases of the nursing process—diagnosis, planning, implementation, and evaluation.

Types of Data

Four types of data are collected by the nurse during assessment—subjective, objective, historical, and current. A complete and accurate data base usually includes a combination of these types.

Subjective data might be described as the individual's view of a situation or a series of events. This information cannot be determined by the nurse independent of interaction or communication with the individual. Subjective data are frequently obtained during the nursing history and include the client's perceptions, feelings, and ideas about self and personal health status. Examples include the client's descriptions of pain, weakness, frustration, nausea, or embarrassment. Information supplied by sources other than the client—e.g., family, consultants, and other members of the health team—may also be subjective if based on the individual's opinion rather than substantiated by fact.

In contrast, objective data are both observable and measurable. This information is usually obtained through the senses—sight, smell, hearing, and touch—during the physical examination of the client. Examples of objective data include respiratory rate, blood pressure, edema, and weight.

During the assessment of a client, the nurse must consider both subjective and objective findings. Frequently, they substantiate each other, as in the case of John Thomas, the client whose incision opened three days after surgery. The subjective information provided by Mr. Thomas, "feels like my stitches are popping," was validated by the nurse's objective findings—pallor, diaphoresis, hypotension, and protrusion of the bowel through the incision.

In the case of Peggy Malletts, the nurse observes the client crying as she stands in front of the nursery two days after premature delivery of her first child. The nurse suggests that Peggy seems "upset," and the client validates that she is "afraid that her baby might die." Here, the objective data observed by the nurse (crying) were substantiated by subjective data obtained from the client (feelings of fear).

At times, subjective and objective data may be in conflict. Juan, a sixteen year old client, denied that he was in pain after surgical repair of an inguinal hernia. Juan's denial would be considered subjective data, since it reflects his feelings of pain. However, the nurse documented several objective findings that are consistent with the usual response to pain (facial grimaces, elevated pulse rate, clutching incision area). In this case the subjective and objective data are in conflict; therefore the nurse must accumulate additional information to resolve the discrepancy.

Another consideration when describing data concerns the element of time. In this context, data may be either historical or current (Bellack and Bamford, 1984). Historical data involve information about events that have occurred prior to the present, which might include previous hospitalizations, normal elimination patterns, or chronic diseases. In contrast, current data refer to events that are occurring in the present—blood pressure, vomiting, postoperative pain. Again, a combination of both current and historical data may be used to verify problems or to identify discrepancies.

Example. A public health nurse visits John Kelly, age 62, at his home following his discharge from an extended care facility. During the initial interview, Mr. Kelly indicates that he has not moved his bowels for two days. When the nurse expresses concern, the client indicates that his normal pattern is every three days.

In this case, the current data (no BM for two days) are invalidated as a problem in view of the historical data (normal pattern every third day).

Example. Kelly O'Keefe, age five, is admitted for a tonsillectomy. In the immediate postoperative period, her pulse rate ranges from 90 to 108. Four hours later, the nurse observes that Kelly is swallowing frequently and her pulse is 124.

In this situation, current data (pulse rate 124) substantiate the existence of a problem (bleeding) when compared with historical data (pulse rate 90 to 108).

For the data base to be complete, the nurse should collect all four types of data. Subjective and objective data provide specific information regarding the client's health status and help to identify problems. Additionally, current and historical data assist in this process by establishing time frames or usual behavioral patterns.

The following exercises are designed to assist you to recognize subjective, objective, historical, and current data.

2–1 TEST YOURSELF

TYPES OF DATA

The following is a list of data. Indicate by checking (✔) whether each item is subjective or objective.

Data	Subjective	Objective
1. "I feel tired today."		
2. Blood pressure 180/96		
3. Speaks only when spoken to		
4. "She seems nervous."		
5. "My leg hurts."		
6. Dirt under nails		
7. Rash on flank		
8. "I need help."		
9. Absent bowel sounds		
10. Respiratory rate 24		

Now, identify each of the following as historical or current.

Data	Historical	Current
1. No prior surgery		
2. "I used to eat when I was nervous."		
3. Temperature 97.8°F		
4. "I'm allergic to sulfa."		
5. Weight 118 lb		
6. Smoked three packs of cigarettes a day until last month		
7. Warm, dry skin		
8. Worked part-time until one year ago		
9. Two episodes of nocturia six months ago		
10. Diminished breath sounds at base of right lung		

2–1 TEST YOURSELF □ ANSWERS

The following is a list of data. Indicate by checking (✔) whether each item is subjective or objective.

Data	Subjective	Objective
1. "I feel tired today."	✔	
2. Blood pressure 180/96		✔
3. Speaks only when spoken to		✔
4. "She seems nervous."	✔	
5. "My leg hurts."	✔	
6. Dirt under nails		✔
7. Rash on flank		✔
8. "I need help."	✔	
9. Absent bowel sounds		✔
10. Respiratory rate 24		✔

Now, identify each of the following items as historical or current.

Data	Historical	Current
1. No prior surgery	✔	
2. "I used to eat when I was nervous."	✔	
3. Temperature 97.8°		✔
4. "I'm allergic to sulfa."		✔
5. Weight 118 lb		✔
6. Smoked three packs of cigarettes a day until last month	✔	
7. Warm, dry skin		✔
8. Worked part-time until one year ago	✔	
9. Two episodes of nocturia six months ago	✔	
10. Diminished breath sounds at base of right lung		✔

Sources of Data

During the assessment phase, data are collected from a variety of sources. These sources are classified as either primary or secondary. The client is the primary source and should be utilized to obtain pertinent subjective data. The client can most accurately (1) share personal perceptions and feelings about health and illness, (2) identify individual goals or problems, and (3) validate responses to diagnostic or treatment modalities.

Secondary sources are those other than the client. These are utilized in situations in which the client is unable to participate or when additional information is required to clarify or validate data supplied by the client. Secondary sources might include the client's family or significant other, individuals in the client's immediate environment, other members of the health team, and the medical record. Family, friends, and coworkers may also provide pertinent historical data regarding the client's normal patterns in the home, at work, and in recreational environments.

Example. Cathy Johnson, age 24, is admitted to the Intensive Care Unit following an automobile accident. Since Cathy is comatose, the nurse interviews her father. During this conversation, Mr. Johnson indicates that Cathy was hit in the eye when she was 13 and has a permanently dilated right pupil.

In this situation, the information obtained from the client's family provides historical data that clarify the nurse's physical findings. These are significant in view of the client's history.

Other members of the health team may also contribute significant data.

☐ Other nurses who have cared for the client during hospitalization may provide information concerning that client's responses.
☐ The physical therapist may be able to assist the nurse to compare the motor skills demonstrated by the client during therapy with those observed on the nursing unit.
☐ The physician may be able to describe the client's emotional response to a previous heart attack.

Each of these secondary sources may add to the nurse's knowledge base and therefore expand the data available for comparing and evaluating client responses.

The individuals in the client's immediate hospital environment may also provide additional information. Visitors may substantiate the nurse's view that the client is less communicative today than on a previous day. Other clients may be able to provide current data that document events that occur when the nurse is not present. For example, the client in another bed may validate the nurse's impression that an elderly client climbed over the siderails and fell out of bed.

The medical record contains an abundance of demographic data—marital status, occupation, religion, insurance. This provides insight into the client's socioeconomic status. Additionally, the record contains current and historical data documented by personnel in other disciplines (physician, dietician, respiratory therapist, social worker, discharge planner). Diagnostic data are also available, including laboratory and radiological findings.

The nurse must carefully consider the client's rights to privacy and confidentiality when obtaining information from secondary sources. Additionally, these client rights may outweigh the needs of others to obtain sensitive data.

Example. Mr. Turi's employer brings him to the emergency department after he vomits blood while at work. The client tells the nurse that he has been drinking a fifth of Scotch a day for five years. While providing information to the nurse, Mr. Turi's employer states, "He drinks, doesn't he? That's why he's bleeding again!"

In this situation, the client's employer is attempting to obtain confidential information about the client's drinking patterns. The nurse should protect the client's privacy by tactfully focusing the conversation on other topics rather than confirm Mr. Turi's alcoholism without his approval.

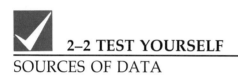

2–2 TEST YOURSELF

SOURCES OF DATA

Case Study

Mr. Ted Alexander, a 50 year old white divorced resident of Las Vegas, was on a business trip to Atlantic City when he developed pain in the right lower abdominal quadrant. He took Alka-Seltzer but obtained little relief, and the pain persisted for the next two days. He was busy with appointments during the day and evening and was able to ignore the pain. He ate very little and took two sleeping pills at night. On the afternoon of the third day, the pain became much more intense, and when it continued for several hours and he began to vomit repeatedly, he went to the emergency department.

Physical examination and laboratory data at this time revealed an alert, well-groomed male with generalized abdominal tenderness, rigidity of the abdominal wall, presence of a palpable mass in the right inguinal area, absent bowel sounds, and a white blood count (WBC) of 20,000/mm³ (normal = 5000–9000). The diagnosis of ruptured appendix was made. He was admitted to the hospital for initial medical management with surgery anticipated at a later date.

Your examination of the patient reveals the following: B/P 140/80, P 116, R 26, T 101.2°F. The patient indicates that he is 6'2" tall and weighs 196 lb. He is alert and oriented and states "My gut is killing me." His skin is warm to the touch and slightly diaphoretic. The patient states that he had been a heavy drinker for 15 years and was admitted to the hospital with cirrhosis two years ago by his family doctor, Dr. Martland, but has never had surgery. He denies drinking for the past two years but smokes two packs of cigarettes daily.

Mr. Alexander is tense throughout your conversation but shares a number of concerns with you, including his separation from his two teenage children who live with him. He is also anxious about being cared for by an unfamiliar physician. The emergency department (ED) nurse indicates that he wears contact lenses and is concerned because he has left his case and supplies as well as his glasses in his hotel. He gives you $750.00 in cash and traveler's checks to deposit in the hospital safe. He has a partial lower plate of dentures and caps on his four front teeth. Further inquiry reveals that the patient prefers a low fat diet, occasionally uses laxatives, and has had several occurrences of urinary urgency and nocturia in the last six months.

The physician states that his treatment plan includes gastric suction, antibiotics, and IV fluid therapy with electrolytes and vitamins until the patient is stabilized enough for exploratory surgery. Mr. Alexander agrees to this plan but is concerned about his job demands and wonders how he will deal with "getting back home when all of this is over."

Based on the case study, identify three examples each of subjective, objective, current, and historical data as well as three secondary sources of data.

Subjective data

1.

2.

3.

Objective data

1.

2.

3.

Current data

1.

2.

3.

Historical data

1.

2.

3.

Secondary sources

1.

2.

3.

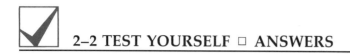

2–2 TEST YOURSELF □ ANSWERS

Subjective data
1. Abdominal pain
2. Height and weight; concerns about separation from children and private MD
3. Low fat diet preference; smoking
Objective data
1. Abdominal rigidity, inguinal mass, absent bowel sounds
2. B/P 140/80, P 116, R 26, T 101.2°F, skin warm and diaphoretic, WBC 20,000/mm³
3. Partial dentures, caps
Current data
1. Vital signs
2. Skin warm, diaphoretic
3. Smokes two packs of cigarettes daily
Historical data
1. Drinking heavily for 15 years
2. No previous surgery; occasional use of laxatives
3. Urgency and nocturia in last six months; pain for two days
Secondary sources
1. Laboratory data
2. Emergency department nurse
3. Physician

Methods of Data Collection

There are three major methods that are utilized to gather information during a nursing assessment. These include interview, observation, and physical examination. These techniques provide the nurse with a logical, systematic approach to the collection of data required for subsequent nursing diagnosis and care planning.

Interview. The interview serves four purposes in the context of a nursing assessment: (1) it allows the nurse to acquire specific information required for diagnosis and planning; (2) it facilitates the nurse-client relationship by creating an opportunity for dialogue; (3) it allows the client to receive information and to participate in identification of problems and goal-setting; and (4) it assists the nurse to determine areas for specific investigation during the other components of the assessment process.

The nursing interview is a complex process that requires refined communication and interaction skills. It differs from the types of interviews performed by other members of the health team since it focuses on identification of client responses that may be treated through nursing intervention. It is a purposeful process designed to allow both nurse and client to give and receive information.

The interview consists of three segments—introduction, body, and closure.

Introduction. In the introductory phase, nurse and client begin to develop a therapeutic relationship. The nurse's professional attitude is probably the most significant factor in creating an environment in which a positive relationship can be developed. The nurse's approach should convey respect for the client; therefore it is appropriate to share introductions. The client should be addressed by name—e.g., "Mr. Jones" rather than "Bill" or "Pop." The nurse should explain the purpose of the interview, estimate the time required, and assess for factors that may inhibit involvement (e.g., pain, lack of privacy). All questions should be directed to the client. Family and other secondary sources should be utilized only when the client is unable to respond. The client should be assured that the information gathered is confidential. These approaches create an atmosphere of trust and sensitivity in which the client may feel comfortable sharing information of a personal nature.

Body. During this second part of the interview, the nurse focuses the dialogue on specific areas designed to obtain the data required. This usually begins with the client's chief complaint and generally incorporates other areas such as past medical history, family history, and religious and cultural data. A more complete listing is seen in Table 2–1.

Interviews are done in a variety of settings, including the hospital, clinic, nursing home, physician's office, home health agency, and client's home. The format for collecting the health history is dependent on the type of setting and the purpose of the interview. Some nurses prefer to use a free-flow approach that begins with the client's chief complaint and extends to other areas based on individual client cues (Figure 2–1). Others prefer a more structured approach that utilizes a specific format. Content areas are defined, and the nurse utilizes a form as a checklist to ensure that all content areas have been addressed (Figure 2–2). The nurse should use the format that is found to be most comfortable and that results in a logical, systematic accumulation of pertinent information about the client.

Closure. The final phase of the interview is closure. During this phase, the nurse prepares the client for termination of the interview. "Mrs. Black, we'll be finishing in a few minutes." The nurse should not introduce new material at this time; however, the client may want to discuss additional topics. If time allows, this may be accomplished, or the nurse may suggest a second interview at another time. The most significant points discussed during the interview should be summarized. This allows the client to verify or negate the nurse's perceptions of major problems, client concerns, and other pertinent data. This also lays the foundation for clarification and mutual goal-setting in the planning process. The nurse should attempt to end the interview in a manner that conveys warmth and

TABLE 2-1 □ **HEALTH HISTORY CONTENT**

Client Profile
Brief statement about the client
Chief Complaint
Client's statement about reason for seeking medical assistance
History of Present Illness
Description of client's symptoms, including onset, location, duration, quality, intensity, aggravating, alleviating, and associated factors, course of illness, problem
Past Medical History
Summary of client's health, including major and minor adult illnesses, previous hospitalization and surgery, major injuries or accidents, drug or food allergies, usual response to illness
Family History
Identification of family members and health trends, including age, sex, and health status of living family members; age, sex, and cause of death of deceased family members; familial history of cancer, heart disease, hypertension, stroke, epilepsy, renal disorders, diabetes, arthritis, tuberculosis
Medication History
Listing of medications, including name, dosage, frequency of administration, duration of therapy, time of last dose (should include nonprescription drugs taken, including aspirin, laxatives, antihistamines, etc.)
Alcohol, Tobacco, and Drug History
Description of usual patterns of usage, including alcohol type, average consumption; tobacco type, amount per day, age started, stopped; drug type, frequency of use
Social History
Summary of employment, occupation, education, hobbies, living environment, recreation, religion
Patterns of Daily Living
Identification of client's usual patterns, including sleep/rest, hygiene, activity, elimination, diet/fluids, health practices

---

appreciation. "Mrs. Black, thanks for sharing this information about yourself—it will be very useful in helping us to plan your care." This may set the scene for future nurse-client interactions throughout their therapeutic relationship.

Factors Affecting the Interview. There are a number of variables that affect the success of a nurse-client interview. These include environmental factors, interviewing techniques, and verbal and nonverbal communication.

ENVIRONMENTAL FACTORS. An informative interview is dependent upon effective nurse-client interaction. The environment in which the interview takes place frequently affects the ability of the client and the nurse to participate in this process. The nurse can attempt to control the environment by manipulating several physical factors.

The interview area should be arranged to allow comfortable face-to-face interaction between the nurse and the client or family. The client should be positioned comfortably in bed or a chair with the nurse seated opposite. Standing over the client should be avoided if possible, since this may convey superiority, disinterest, or haste.

Privacy should be assured, since the client is expected to answer many personal questions. This may be accomplished by pulling a curtain, finding a quiet spot, or closing a door. Privacy also increases the potential for accurate, complete information and assists in creating a trusting relationship. To facilitate the concentration of both nurse and client, the interview area should be free from noise, odors, and interruptions. The temperature of the area should be comfortable, and lighting should allow both participants to observe each other clearly.

NURSING ASSESSMENT FORM

Name _____ Age _____ Date _____

Prefers to be called _____ Assessment made by _____ RN

Areas	Subjective/Objective Data

Client Perceptions of:

   Current health status
   Goals
   Needed/usable services

Functional Abilities:

   Breathing/circulation
   Elimination
   Emotional/cognitive
   Mobility/safety
   Nutrition
   Hygiene/grooming
   Sensory input
   Sexuality
   Sleep/rest

Resources/Support Systems:

   Environmental
   Personal/social
   Other

Figure 2–1 □ Sample free-flow nursing assessment form. (From Carnevali, D.: Nursing Care Planning. 3rd ed. Philadelphia: J. B. Lippincott, 1983.)

MERCER MEDICAL CENTER
NURSING HISTORY AND PHYSICAL

Date _____ Time _____ A.M.
                                                               P.M.
BP _____ TPR _____

Admitting Diagnosis _____
_____

PAST MEDICAL HISTORY (medical, surgical, trauma)

Height _____ Weight _____
ALLERGIES AND REACTIONS _____

MEDICATIONS Name & Dosage	Usual Time Taken	Time of Last Dose

REASONS FOR HOSPITALIZATION (onset, character, methods used to resolve problem)
_____
_____
_____

Signature_____

COMMUNICATION

SUBJECTIVE   OBJECTIVE
☐ Hearing Loss   Comments: _____   ☐ Glasses   ☐ Language Barrier
☐ Visual Changes _____   ☐ Contact Lens   ☐ Hearing Aide
☐ Denied   _____   R   L
                 _____   Pupil Size _____ ☐ Speech Difficulties
                 _____   Reaction _____

OXYGENATION

☐ Dyspnea   Comments: _____   Resp   ☐ Regular   ☐ Irregular
☐ Smoking History _____   Describe:_____
_____ _____
☐ Cough   _____
☐ Sputum   _____   R _____
☐ Denied   _____   L _____

CIRCULATION

☐ Chest Pain   Comments: _____   Heart Rhythm ☐ Regular   ☐ Irregular
☐ Leg Pain   _____   Ankle Edema _____
☐ Numbness of   _____
  Extremities   _____   Pulse   Car.   Rad.   DP   Fem.*
☐ Denied   _____   R _____
                                         L _____
                                         Comments: _____

                                         *If applicable

NUTRITION

Diet: _____   ☐ Dentures   ☐ None
☐ N   ☐ V   Comments: _____   Full   Partial   With Patient
Character   _____
☐ Recent change in _____   Upper   ☐   ☐   ☐
  weight, appetite _____
☐ Swallowing   _____   Lower   ☐   ☐   ☐
  difficulty   _____
☐ Denied   _____

RBG 13122 (11/84)

Figure 2–2 ☐ Sample structured nursing assessment form. (Courtesy of Mercer Medical Center, Trenton, NJ.)

Illustration continued on opposite page

	SUBJECTIVE		OBJECTIVE		
ELIMINATION	Usual bowel pattern	☐ Urinary Frequency	Comments: _____	Bowel Sounds _____	
	☐ Constipation Remedy	☐ Urgency ☐ Dysuria ☐ Hematuria		Abdominal distention present: ☐ Yes ☐ No	
	Date of last BM	☐ Incontinence ☐ Polyuria		Urine* (color, consistency, odor)	
	☐ Diarrhea Character	☐ Foley in place ☐ Denied		*If foley in place	
MGT. OF HEALTH AND ILLNESS	☐ Alcohol ☐ Denied (Amount, frequency)		Briefly describe patient's ability to follow treatments (diet, meds, etc.) for chronic health problems (if present).		
	☐ BSE Last Pap Smear _____ LMP: _____				
SKIN INTEGRITY	☐ Dry ☐ Itching ☐ Other ☐ Denied *Use Skin/body Stamp on Progress Notes	Comments: _____	☐ Dry ☐ Flushed ☐ Moist	☐ Cold ☐ Warm ☐ Cyanotic	☐ Pale
			*Rashes, ulcers, decubitus (describe size, location, drainage)		
ACTIVITY/SAFETY	☐ Convulsions ☐ Dizziness ☐ Limited motion of joints Limitations in ability to: ☐ Ambulate ☐ Bathe self ☐ Other ☐ Denied	Comments: _____	☐ LOC and Orientation _____ Gait: ☐ Walker ☐ Cane ☐ Other ☐ Steady ☐ Unsteady _____ ☐ Sensory and motor losses in face or extremities _____ ☐ ROM limitations _____		
COMFORT SLEEP/WAKE	☐ Pain (Location, frequency, remedies) ☐ Nocturia ☐ Sleep Difficulties ☐ Denied	Comments: _____	☐ Facial Grimaces ☐ Guarding ☐ Other signs of pain _____ ☐ Siderail release form signed (60 + years)		
COPING	Occupation _____ Members of household _____ Most supportive person _____		Observed non-verbal behavior _____ Person and phone number that can be reached at any time		
	R.N. Signature _____				

Figure 2–2 *Continued*

INTERVIEWING TECHNIQUES. Interviews are most informative when the nurse utilizes both verbal and nonverbal techniques to obtain data. The combination of both approaches facilitates the acquisition of an accurate, complete data base.

Verbal Techniques. The most commonly used verbal techniques include questioning, reflection, and supplementary statements. The nurse who uses all of these approaches during the interview is more likely to be successful in obtaining the most significant information from the client.

Questioning allows the nurse to obtain information from the client, clarify perceptions of client responses, and validate other subjective or objective data. Questions may be open, closed, or biased.

Open questions are those that by their nature elicit the client's perception of an event or description of concerns or feelings. Generally, these questions require more than a one or two word response.

Examples

"What happened today that made you come to the emergency department?"

"How did you feel when the doctor told you about your blood pressure?"

"Which medications do you take on a regular basis?"

"What do you usually do when the pain occurs?"

Questions beginning with "what," "how," or "which" tend to result in the most detailed client response. "Why" questions tend to put the client in a defensive position.

Examples

"Why did you do that?"

"Why didn't you see a doctor sooner?"

The following outlines the advantages and disadvantages of open questions.

Advantages	Disadvantages
☐ Provide clients with the stimulus to express important concerns	☐ Tend to elicit lengthy or wordy responses in a limited time frame
☐ Help to facilitate communication by encouraging clients to respond	☐ Allow the client to stray from content of question or focus on irrelevant topics (particularly when client is not comfortable discussing topic)
☐ Tend to be less threatening and to elicit more honest replies	

Closed questions are those that require brief one or two word responses. They are used most frequently to obtain specific facts.

Examples

"Did you take your blood pressure medicine today?"
"How long did the pain last?"
"When was your last menstrual period?"
"How many times did you have diarrhea yesterday?"

Advantages	Disadvantages
□ Avoid lengthy responses □ Allow the nurse to focus the interview □ Help to clarify responses to open-ended questions	□ Discourage verbalization and limit the type and amount of data obtained (brief and superficial) □ Tend to make the client feel defensive

Example

Nurse:	What do you usually do when the back pain occurs? (Open)
Client:	Well, I usually lie down and take two pain pills.
Nurse:	Did you do that today before you came to the hospital? (Closed)
Client:	Yes.

Biased questions are those that tend to elicit a specific response or reaction from a client. They may be either open or closed. The most commonly used are leading or loaded questions. Leading questions imply that a particular response is preferred. Clients tend to answer these questions with responses they feel are desirable.

Examples

"You don't take drugs, do you?"
"There's no history of mental illness in your family, is there?"
"You're feeling better today, aren't you?"

Loaded questions are used to elicit the client's reaction to a specific topic. The nurse is usually trying to evaluate the client's nonverbal response more than the content of the actual reply to the question.

Examples

"Do you think that your pain increases after your husband visits?"
"Does your drinking interfere with your work?"

When asking questions of this nature, the nurse is watching for squirming, lack of eye contact, or other signs of uneasiness. This nonverbal behavior may be more revealing than the client's verbal response. Biased questions tend to intimidate clients and frequently block the communication process. Clients often provide responses that they believe are expected; therefore, the information may be inaccurate. Biased questions should be used only when other techniques have been unsuccessful. Ideally, the use of a mixture of open and closed questioning will result in accurate, complete data, eliminating the need for biased questions.

The second verbal interviewing technique is the use of *reflection*. The nurse's perception of the client's response is repeated or rephrased. Repetition encourages the client to continue discussion of a particular area of content. The nurse repeats key words from the client's statement and assists the client to explore the topic more completely.

Example

Nurse:	How did you feel when the doctor told you about your high blood pressure?
Client:	I was really afraid.
Nurse:	You were really afraid? (Repetition of key words)
Client:	Yes, I thought I might have a stroke and die or be an invalid.

Since rephrasing provides the client with the nurse's interpretation of the information discussed, this allows both nurse and client to expand, clarify, or correct the nurse's perception.

Example

Client:	I found this lump in my breast last week when I was taking a shower. My mother had them too before she died from cancer.
Nurse:	You're afraid that you might have cancer?
Client:	Yes. I'm too young to die; my children need me.

In this case the nurse's perceptions were verified by the client.

Example

Client:	I never had this dizziness or nausea until the doctor started me on that new blood pressure medicine.
Nurse:	You think that the medicine is the cause of the problems you're having now?
Client:	No, not really, but I think it may be part of the problem.

Here, the client clarified the nurse's interpretation of the initial statement.

After reflective statements, clients may seek advice or reassurance or ask the nurse to validate their feelings. The client might respond with

"What do you think?" "It's OK, isn't it?" or "What would you do?" Such responses may also be the client's attempt to obtain additional information. The nurse should avoid providing advice, unrealistic reassurance, or opinions since this tends to shift the accountability for decision-making from the client to the nurse. The most effective method of dealing with this type of interaction is to use reflection to redirect the question.

Example

>Client: The doctor told me that I can either have my hysterectomy the day after tomorrow or go home and come back in six weeks. What would you do, nurse?
>
>Nurse: You're not sure whether you should have the surgery now or later? Let's look at the pros and cons of each.

This approach allowed the nurse to (1) rephrase the client's concerns, (2) clarify the decision that needed to be made by the client, and (3) create an environment that would encourage the client to look at her options objectively before making a decision.

The use of *supplementary statements* may encourage the client to continue verbalization throughout the interview. Short phrases such as "um-hm," "yes," "go on," "I see," and "what happened next?" send a clear message. These brief responses let the client know that the nurse is interested and frequently stimulate further communication. They are particularly effective when accompanied by nonverbal cues such as touch, eye contact, and nodding the head.

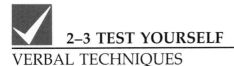 **2–3 TEST YOURSELF**

VERBAL TECHNIQUES

Read the following statements and identify them as open (O), closed (C), biased (B), reflective (R), or supplementary (S).

_____"When did you first notice the lump in your breast?"

_____"And then?"

_____"You don't really believe that old wives' tale, do you?"

_____"You're confused about how many times a day you should be taking this pill?"

_____"How do you know when your blood sugar is low?"

_____"When did you stop beating your wife?"

_____"Oh, when you went to India you got malaria?"

_____"What do you think you can do to assist in your recovery?"

_____"Do you have any questions about what will be happening to you tomorrow?"

_____"Go on."

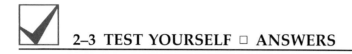

2–3 TEST YOURSELF □ ANSWERS

Key—(O) open, (C) closed, (B) biased, (R) reflective, (S) supplementary
(C)   "When did you first notice the lump in your breast?"
(S)   "And then?"
(B)   "You don't really believe that old wives' tale, do you?"
(R)   "You're confused about how many times a day you should be taking this pill?"
(O)   "How do you know when your blood sugar is low?"
(B)   "When did you stop beating your wife?"
(R)   "Oh, when you went to India you got malaria?"
(O)   "What do you think you can do to assist in your recovery?"
(C)   "Do you have any questions about what will be happening to you tomorrow?"
(S)   "Go on."

Nonverbal Techniques. The nurse should be aware of a number of nonverbal methods that may facilitate or enhance communication during the interview. The nonverbal components of a nurse-client interaction frequently convey a message more effectively than the actual spoken words. In fact, if the verbal and nonverbal messages differ, the nonverbal message tends to be accepted more readily. The most common nonverbal components include facial expression, body position, touch, voice, silence, and active listening.

The client's *facial expressions* often reveal important information. The nurse should watch for appropriateness of expression, frowning, and lack of eye contact.

Appropriateness of expression suggests that facial expression should be congruent with the words being spoken and the context of the conversation. The nurse should be particularly alert to situations in which the expression on the client's face does not match the verbal message. For example, when a client describes himself as depressed, the nurse would not expect to see a smile on his face. Similarly, when a woman talks about how happy she is in her marriage, her facial expression usually indicates sincerity. The nurse might question this sincerity if her statement is accompanied by a smirk.

The nurse should also be concerned if the facial expression is not appropriate to the context of the message. For example, sometimes a nurse will encounter a client who smiles when discussing a serious problem. The smile, which may be resulting from uneasiness, could mislead the nurse into believing that the client is not concerned about the problem.

Frowning may indicate disagreement, lack of understanding, pain, anger, or unhappiness. For example, when a nurse is explaining to Mrs. Kuroishi that she should take her pulse each day before taking her digoxin, the client frowns. The nurse might interpret this as an indication of unwillingness to carry out this step. In reality, Mrs. Kuroishi does not know how to take her pulse.

Lack of eye contact may mean that the client is uncomfortable, shy, nonassertive, bored, intimidated, or withdrawn. For example, in a vene- real disease clinic, the nurse frequently questions clients about sexual contacts. In response to this question, Tyrell Williams turns his face away. The nurse might interpret this change in eye contact as embarrassment. In reality, Tyrell is trying to remember a number of names.

The nurse may want to clarify discrepancies between facial expres- sions and verbal messages or context. For example, the nurse might say, "I notice that you are smiling when you discuss your illness, but your words indicate your concern. I'm confused. Could you clarify this for me?"

Similarly, facial expressions exhibited by the nurse may also convey mixed messages. For example, the nurse who smiles inappropriately when the client shares very personal or sensitive information may upset the client. In fact, the nurse may feel uncomfortable discussing the topic. Likewise, frowning after a client's comments may be seen as being judgmental, when in reality the nurse may have a headache. Lack of eye contact because of preoccupation with a confused client in the other bed may be interpreted as lack of interest.

Body position and stance are elements of interaction that convey a nonverbal message. The nurse should attempt to create an environment of warmth and trust. This is frequently accomplished by a calm, relaxed posture. This communicates interest and caring and tends to help the client feel comfortable in disclosing personal information. A hurried approach, an inappropriately warm or cold attitude, a rigid or overly casual posture communicate disinterest, boredom, or preoccupation. These nonverbal messages tend to confuse the client and inhibit the interview process.

The nurse should observe the nonverbal messages communicated by the client's posture or stance throughout the interview. The timing of specific behaviors may be particularly significant. A relaxed posture may indicate readiness to share information, just as a tense or rigid stance suggests unwillingness to share, pain, or anxiety. The relaxed client who tenses or shifts position when discussing family relationships or alcohol consumption may be communicating discomfort in discussing particularly sensitive information.

Gestures may also provide the nurse with information about the client.

Finger pointing		anger; control
Hand wringing		anxiety
Nodding	*may suggest*	agreement
Shoulder shrugging		uncertainty

The nurse should be particularly observant for discrepancies between the client's spoken words and the nonverbal messages communicated by posture or stance.

The use of *touch* may also significantly affect the interview process. The individual's use of or response to touch may effectively communicate specific attitudes, feelings, or responses. Clients may vary in their degree of comfort with touching or being touched. The nurse's use of touch should be determined by the client's readiness to accept it. This is frequently evidenced by response to an introductory handshake or to the touching that accompanies taking a pulse or blood pressure. The client's tolerance of touch may be dependent upon cultural background, social maturity, and past experiences. Some clients consider even simple touch an intrusion, and withdrawal from touch may be demonstrating fear, pain, or resentment. On the other hand, the client who grasps the nurse's arm, squeezes hands, or touches the face may be communicating warmth, appreciation, or the need for support or reassurance.

The nurse may convey caring, concern, and support by a simple touch on the client's arm, squeezing of a hand, or an arm around the shoulder. Similarly, rough, rushed, or insincere touch communicates the opposite message.

Although *voice* is usually considered to be a verbal technique, it will be discussed here because of the nonverbal messages that may be conveyed. There are a number of vocal characteristics that may be significant in determining the perceptions of both nurse and client. These include tone of voice, rate of speech, and volume. The nurse who speaks calmly, relatively slowly, and at a comfortable level communicates relaxation, patience, and concern with privacy. The client may be intimidated, embarrassed, or uncomfortable when interviewed by the overly excited nurse who is loud or speaks too rapidly.

The client who speaks slowly, in a monotone, or with a flat affect may be worried or depressed. Conversely, loud or rapid speech suggests anger, pain, impatience, or hearing deficits. These may be particularly significant if observed at specific points in the interview.

Example

Nurse: How do you feel about your surgery?

Client: I told you, it's nothing to worry about, it's only a cyst. (Spoken loudly, through clenched teeth.)

Clearly this client is communicating some type of distress. It may be anger or impatience in response to repeated questioning or anxiety about the possible outcome of surgery.

There are a number of other sounds that may convey meaning. They may indicate impatience, sarcasm, pain, anxiety, embarrassment, emphasis, agreement, or disagreement.

Nurses and clients are often uncomfortable when periods of *silence* occur during the interview. However, silence may be an important tool for the nurse. It provides an opportunity to (1) review what has transpired up to that point in the interview, (2) collect thoughts, and (3) begin to organize data. Frequently, inexperienced interviewers attempt to fill the gaps in conversation with multiple questions to avoid the discomfort associated with silence. This may communicate anxiety to the client and is often confusing. The client may feel pressured, rushed, or unable to respond.

Silence evidenced by the client may be significant in conveying discomfort, thoughtfulness, or embarrassment. The nurse should consciously avoid filling silent periods too quickly. This indicates an acceptance of the client's feelings and may strengthen the nurse-client relationship.

The verbal and nonverbal components of the interview process communicate vital messages to the participants. The most skilled interviewers use the technique of *active listening* to enhance interaction with clients. This method involves three stages—listening to the verbal component, identifying the existence of nonverbal cues, and carefully determining the significance of both. The nurse who learns to listen not only to what is spoken but also to what is left unsaid is able to interpret the client's feelings and responses effectively and to identify specific areas requiring further exploration. Consequently this (1) allows more accurate reflection of these perceptions to the client, (2) encourages clarification or validation by the client, and (3) promotes the acquisition of a more accurate and complete data base. Table 2–2 summarizes guidelines for interviewing.

Observation. The second method of data collection used during the assessment phase is observation. Systematic observation involves the use of the senses to acquire information about the client, significant other, the environment, and interactions among these three variables. Observation is a skill that requires discipline and practice on the part of the nurse. It demands a broad knowledge base and conscious use of the senses—sight,

TABLE 2–2 □ **GUIDELINES FOR INTERVIEWING**

1. Select the environment carefully, assuring privacy and comfort. Avoid noises, odors, interruptions, inadequate lighting, and temperature extremes.
2. Defer the interview when indicated because of the client's condition or environmental barriers.
3. Create an environment of trust, caring, and concern with a calm unhurried approach.
4. Utilize the client as the primary source of data whenever possible, address by name, and avoid talking around the client to family or others.
5. Begin with introductions, a handshake, and an explanation of the purpose of the interview, including its relationship to nursing care.
6. Use terminology appropriate to the client's level of understanding. Speak clearly and distinctly.
7. Discuss the client's chief complaint early in the interview. Focus on this complaint and determine its effects on the client.
8. Encourage verbalization by using open-ended questions and supportive statements. Discuss general nonthreatening information before asking personal questions. Avoid interruptions, "why" questions, and biased questions.
9. Verify perceptions of the client's responses by using the reflective techniques of repetition and rephrasing.
10. Provide realistic reassurance if necessary. Avoid giving advice, opinions, or unrealistic reassurance.
11. Listen actively, maintain eye contact, and observe the nonverbal behavior of the client.
12. Conclude the interview with a brief summary of the client's problems, including anticipated nursing interventions.
13. Document as soon as possible away from the client's bedside, utilizing notations written briefly during the interview.

smell, hearing, feeling, and taste. Table 2–3 provides a list of the types of observations that can be obtained by the use of the senses.

The observations identified by the senses may be either positive or negative indices in the individual client. For example, crying may be viewed as a positive expression of grief in the parents of a terminally ill child, the odor of perfume may indicate progress in a women after disfiguring breast surgery, or the presence of bowel sounds may signal the return of bowel function following abdominal surgery.

Each of the individual findings identified during observation requires further investigation, which may either substantiate or negate the nurse's initial impressions.

Physical Examination. The third major method of collecting data during the assessment process is physical examination. The focus of the physician's physical exam is the diagnosis of disease. The nurse's examination concentrates on (1) further defining the client's response to the disease process, particularly those amenable to nursing actions, (2) establishing baseline data for comparison in evaluating the efficacy of nursing or medical interventions, and (3) substantiating subjective data obtained during interview or other nurse-client interactions.

Techniques. The nurse uses four specific techniques during the examination—inspection, palpation, percussion, and auscultation.

TABLE 2–3 □ OBSERVATION: USE OF SENSES

Sight

Abrasions, absence of body part, absent or broken teeth, baldness, bandages, bitten nails, bleeding, blinking, blisters, boils, books, braces, bunions, burns, calluses, canes, casts, catheter, cleanliness of client or environment, clenched fists, clothing, convulsions, corns, crusting, crutches, crying, cyanosis, decubitus, dentures, diaphoresis, diarrhea, distention, drainage, drooling, ecchymosis, edema, eyeglasses, feces, fidgeting, fistula, flaking, flared nares, flies, flowers, frowning, gait, hangnail, hearing aids, hives, intravenous device, jaundice, jewelry, lighting, make-up, moles, monitor electrodes, mottling, newspaper, ostomy, paresis, petechiae, pimples, position—sitting, standing, or lying, posture, pregnancy, ptosis, purulent drainage, redness, room—type, size, and temperature, scabs, scars, scratches, scratching, shivering, significant other, skin color, slings, sneezing, squinting, stairs, sternal retraction, striae, support stockings, tatoo, telephone, television, tension, toilet articles, twitching, ulcerations, urine, vaccination, varicosities, vomiting, walker, warts, wheelchair, yawning

Hearing

Banging, barking, blood pressure, bruit, burping, clicking, coughing, crying, dripping, eructation, esophageal speech, expressions of pain, anger, sorrow, or depression, gargling, gasping, groaning, grunting, gurgling, harsh cough, heart rate and rhythm, hiccough, hissing, hoarseness, hyperactive or hypoactive bowel sounds, knocking, laughing, loudness, moaning, panting, radio, scratching, screaming, sighing, sirens, sneezing, squeaking, stammering, stuttering, sucking, telephone ringing, television, tone of voice, wheezing, whispering, whistling, yawning

Touch

Coarseness, coldness, dryness, edema, goose bumps, hardness, heat, lumps, masses, moisture, pain, pulsation, relaxation, roughness, skin texture, smoothness, softness, subcutaneous emphysema, swelling, tautness, temperature, tension, tremors, warmth, wetness

Smell

Alcohol, axillary odor, bleeding, breath or body odor, disinfectants, feces, flowers, foot odor, garlic, gas, hair spray, marijuana, medicine, onion, perfume, perspiration, pubic odor, purulent drainage, tobacco, urine, vomitus

Inspection refers to the visual examination of the client to determine normal, unusual, or abnormal conditions or responses. It is a type of observation that focuses on specific behaviors or physical features. Inspection is also more systematic and detailed than observation, since it specifies characteristics such as size, shape, position, anatomical location, color, texture, appearance, movement, and symmetry.

Generally, inspection refers to the use of the unaided eye; however, the expanded role of the nurse in a variety of settings may incorporate the use of instruments. Those used most frequently are the otoscope and ophthalmoscope. These tools allow the nurse to complete a more comprehensive and accurate examination of the eye or ear when indicated.

Palpation is the use of touch to determine the characteristics of body structure under the skin. This technique allows the nurse to evaluate size, shape, texture, temperature, moisture, pulsation, vibration, consistency, and mobility. The nurse's hands are the tools of palpation, and specific parts are utilized to assess particular characteristics. The back of the hand is most useful in assessing temperature because the skin in this area is thinner and allows discrimination of temperature differences. The fingertips are used to determine texture and size, since nerve endings are concentrated there. The palmar surfaces of the metacarpal joints are the most sensitive to vibration and therefore are particularly useful in detecting phenomena such as thrills over the heart or peristalsis.

Light palpation is the method used to examine most body parts. The use of the nurse's dominant hand is preferred. The hand is held parallel to the body part being examined, with fingers extended. Gentle pressure is exerted downward while the nurse moves the hand in a circular motion. This technique is frequently used in breast examination to detect the presence and characteristics of abnormal masses. Deep palpation is particularly effective when examining the abdomen to locate organs or identify unusual masses. This technique requires both hands, one for pressure application and the other as a sensor. The nurse's dominant hand is placed over the area to be palpated and becomes the passive sensor. The other hand is positioned on top and is used to apply pressure. The client's facial expression and body movements during palpation provide the nurse with additional information to assist in evaluating variables such as the degree of pain or discomfort.

Percussion involves the nurse's striking of a body surface with a finger or fingers to produce sounds. This allows determination of size, density, organ boundaries, and location. Direct percussion occurs when the nurse strikes or taps the body surface directly with one or more fingers of one hand. This method is often used to define the cardiac border. Indirect percussion is used more frequently. The nurse places the index or middle finger of one hand firmly on the skin and strikes with the middle finger of the other hand.

The sounds resulting from percussion may be described as flat, dull, resonant, or tympanic. Flat sounds are low-pitched and abrupt and are produced when muscle or bone is percussed. Dull sounds are medium-pitched and thudding and may be heard over the liver and spleen. Resonance is a clear, hollow sound produced by percussion over a normal air-filled lung. Tympany is a loud, high-pitched sound heard over a gas-filled stomach or puffed-out cheek.

Auscultation involves listening to the sounds produced by the organs of the body. The nurse may use direct auscultation (with the unaided ear) to detect sounds such as wheezing. Generally, however, sounds are evaluated indirectly by using a stethoscope. This technique is used most frequently to determine the characteristics of lung, heart, and bowel sounds. The nurse identifies the frequency, intensity, quality, and duration of auscultated sounds.

Each of the four techniques—inspection, palpation, percussion, and auscultation—may be performed independently. However, the most effective method of physical examination is a comprehensive approach including a combination of techniques.

Examination Approaches. A systematic methodology is vital to accurate and complete physical examination. There are a variety of useful and practical approaches used by nurses to assess clients systematically. The head-to-toe, major body systems, and functional health patterns approaches are described below.

HEAD-TO-TOE. This approach begins with the client's head and systematically and symmetrically progresses down the body to the feet. The components of the physical examination are outlined in Figure 2–3. A more detailed guide is found in Appendix A.

MAJOR BODY SYSTEMS. In this approach, the nurse examines the body by systems rather than individual body parts. Information from the interview and observation assists the nurse to determine which systems require particular emphasis. The components of this system are identified in Figure 2–4, with a more detailed guide in Appendix B.

FUNCTIONAL HEALTH PATTERNS. This approach allows the nurse to collect data systematically by evaluating the functional health patterns of the client. The nurse attempts to identify patterns and to focus the physical examination on particular functional areas. The list in Table 2–4 identifies the patterns evaluated. A more detailed guide may be found in Appendix C.

Comparison of these approaches reveals that the information obtained is identical. Therefore, the nurse should select the method that is found to be most effective or more appropriate to a particular practice setting.

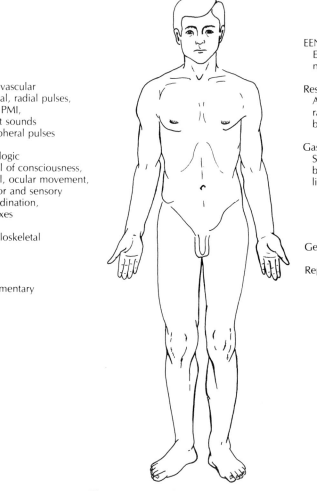

Body Systems Assessment

General Appearance

EENT
  Eyes, ears,
  nose, throat

Respiratory
  Airway, respiratory
  rate, rhythm,
  breath sounds

Gastrointestinal
  Stomach, abdomen,
  bowel sounds,
  liver, spleen

Cardiovascular
  Apical, radial pulses,
  B/P, PMI,
  heart sounds
  peripheral pulses

Neurologic
  Level of consciousness,
  pupil, ocular movement,
  motor and sensory
  coordination,
  reflexes

Musculoskeletal

Genitourinary

Reproductive

Integumentary

Figure 2–3 □ Body systems assessment.

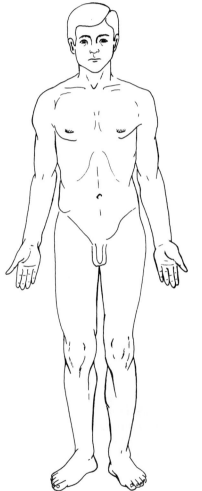

Head–to–Toe Assessment

General Appearance

Vital Signs

Head
Face
Eyes
Ears
Nose
Mouth/throat
Neck

Chest
Lungs
Heart

Abdomen
Kidneys

Genitalia
Rectum

Extremities

Back

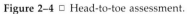

Figure 2–4 □ Head-to-toe assessment.

TABLE 2-4 □ **HEALTH PATTERNS**

Health perception/health management
Nutritional/metabolic
Elimination
Activity/exercise
Sleep/rest
Cognitive/perceptual
Self-perception
Sexuality/sexual functioning
Coping/stress management
Value/belief systems
Physical examination
General appearance
Vital signs, height, weight
Eyes
Mouth
Hearing
Pulses
Respirations
Skin
Functional ability
Mental status

Regardless of the approach selected, skilled physical examination requires discipline and practice to perfect assessment techniques.

In summary, the first component of the assessment phase, data collection, involves the accumulation of subjective, objective, current, and historical information from primary and secondary sources. The nurse utilizes interviewing, observation, and physical examination skills to acquire an organized, accurate, and systematic data base about the individual client.

Documentation

The second component of the assessment phase is documentation of the data base. Although the following discussion of documentation is primarily directed toward the recording of data accumulated during the assessment, documentation is integral to all phases of the nursing process.

Purposes of Documentation

The recording of data in the client's medical record is an important part of the nursing process for a variety of reasons. First, it establishes a mechanism for communication among the members of the health team. This provides a variety of disciplines with pertinent, accurate, and current data about the client as an individual. A common frustration of clients in health systems is repeated questioning and examination by a variety of personnel—physicians, nurses, therapists, dieticians. Complete documentation assists in eliminating this repetition and prevents gaps in data. It also helps to create positive relationships between the client and health care providers.

Second, documentation of assessment data facilitates the delivery of quality client care. The information collected allows the nurse to develop preliminary nursing diagnoses, outcomes, and nursing interventions. Accurately documented baseline findings form the standard for comparison of subsequent data collection, allowing the nurse to validate, clarify, or update preliminary diagnoses and facilitating the provision of consistent individualized care.

Third, documentation assures a mechanism for the evaluation of individual client care. Medical records are reviewed by a variety of internal systems and external regulatory agencies. These may include quality assurance and risk management committees, State Departments of Health (DOH), Professional Review Organizations (PRO), and the Joint Commission on Accreditation of Hospitals (JCAH). These committees and organizations have developed standards for the delivery of nursing care. Careful documentation, beginning with the assessment data base, assists in demonstrating compliance with these accepted standards.

Fourth, documentation creates a permanent legal record of the care provided to the client. Although the medical record is confidential, it is available as a legal document in a number of situations. Obviously, the chart may be utilized to evaluate liability in a malpractice litigation. However, it may also be used to document client competence, determine the extent of injury in accident or compensation claims, or substantiate the provision of specific treatment modalities for reimbursement purposes. Therefore, detailed accurate documentation, beginning with assessment findings, may protect the client, the care providers (particularly nurses), and the institution or agency.

Finally, documentation provides the foundation for nursing research. The information found in the medical record may be utilized as a source for identification of research topics specific to nursing practice. Validation of nursing diagnoses, comparison of client responses to nursing interventions, and development of nurse-client relationships are potential areas of exploration. The accumulation of a body of research associated with nursing practice helps to define nursing as a science and to refine the nursing process.

The documentation of the nursing assessment should clearly identify those findings that necessitate nursing interventions. These include a variety of factors affecting the client's health status or ability to function. The client's responses, perceptions, feelings, and coping mechanisms are particularly significant in the formulation of nursing diagnoses and the identification of specific nursing orders.

Guidelines for Documentation

The format for recording the nursing assessment varies among practice settings. Regardless of the type and structure of the documentation tool, there are some general guidelines that should be considered.

□ 1. The nurse's entries should be written objectively without bias, value judgments, or personal opinion. The subjective information provided by the client, family, and other members of the health team should be included. The nurse should use quotation marks to clearly identify these types of statements.

Example

Client's description of illness: "My diabetes is out of control, and I'm here to have tests and get it regulated."

□ 2. Descriptions or interpretations of objective data should be supported by specific observations.

Example

Emotional status: Depressed, sits in darkened room with curtain pulled around bed, rarely initiates conversation, responds in monotone with short answers when questioned, limited eye contact, cries softly.

These findings support the nurse's interpretation of depression.

□ 3. Generalizations should be avoided, including "basket terms" such as "good," "fair," "usual," "normal." These descriptions are open to broad interpretation based on the reader's point of reference.

Example

"Abdomen moderately distended" may be interpreted differently by each nurse reading the entry. More specific documentation might include exact measurement of abdominal girth.

"Fair mobility" may suggest that the client was able to perform activities of daily living effectively. In reality, the nurse may mean that the client was able to turn independently in bed but required assistance with bathing, feeding, and ambulating.

"Normal bowel patterns" is more clearly defined by "moves bowels every other day without the use of laxatives."

☐ 4. Findings should be described as thoroughly as possible, including defining characteristics such as size and shape.

For example, the description of a client's decubitus ulcer should include measurements, depth, color, odor, and drainage. This is particularly important when documenting the initial assessment, since this information is the base line for evaluating the effectiveness of nursing interventions.

☐ 5. The nurse should document data clearly and concisely, avoiding superfluous information and long, rambling sentences.

Example

"The client indicates that she didn't feel good for five days, so she went to the doctor and told him about her symptoms. He gave her three medications including antihistamine, antibiotic, and cough medicine. These didn't help so she went to the emergency room, and the doctor there admitted her."

This could be reworded as: "History of fever, cough, and nasal congestion × 5 days, unrelieved by antihistamine, antibiotic, antitussives prescribed by family physician."

☐ 6. The assessment should be written or printed legibly in non-erasable ink. Errors in documentation should be corrected in a manner that does not obscure the original entry. The most commonly used method involves drawing a single line through the incorrect item, writing "error," and initialing the entry. The use of white-out, erasure, or crossing out to obliterate the entry is not acceptable.

☐ 7. Entries should be correct in grammar and spelling. The nurse should incorporate only those abbreviations approved for use in the particular practice setting. Slang, clichés, and labels should be avoided except in the context of a direct quotation.

Figure 2–5 demonstrates how the information obtained from Ted Alexander, the man described in 2–2 Test Yourself, would be documented.

COMPUTERS AND NURSING ASSESSMENT

Computer applications that automate all phases of the nursing process have been designed and implemented. These applications include both components of the assessment phase—data collection and documentation.

HAMILTON HOSPITAL
NURSING ADMISSION · ASSESSMENT FORM

TPR 101.8° - 116 - 26   B/P 140/80 Height 6'2" Weight 196 lb
Mode of Admission: Amb. _____ Wch. ✓ Stretcher _____ Clothing Sheet Completed ✓
Admitted From: Admissions _____ E.R. ✓ 2:30 pm

ORIENTATION TO ROOM:
Use of Call Bell ✓   Use of telephone ✓   Hi-low bed ✓
Use of Intercom ✓   Location of bathroom ✓   T.V. rental ✓

ADMISSION DIAGNOSIS: Ruptured Appendix
MENTAL STATUS: Level of consciousness - alert, oriented to person, place, time,
Level of comprehension - responds appropriately, asks questions
PATIENT'S DESCRIPTION OF ILLNESS: "my gut is killing me"

PAST ILLNESS/HOSPITALIZATIONS: Hospitalized 2 years ago in Las Vegas for cirrhosis

FAMILY PHYSICIAN: Dr Maitland (in Nevada) FREQUENCY SEEN: annually & when ill
If no family physician, other type of health care -

ALLERGIES & REACTIONS:
Food None known
Drugs None known
Other None known

MEDICATIONS:

NAME OF DRUG	DOSE	FREQUENCY	HOW LONG TAKEN	LAST DOSE
No meds on a regular basis but has			taken Alka Seltzer	
and over the counter sleeping pills			prior to	
admission for relief of pain				
Occasional use of laxatives				

PROSTHESIS: Glasses at hotel   Contact Lenses in eyes   Artificial Eye no
Dentures partial lower Limbs no   Hearing Aid no
Breast no   OTHER: 4 capped front teeth

PATTERNS OF DAILY LIVING:
Rest/Sleep Sleeps 6-8 hrs, early riser, difficulty sleeping X 2 days, pain due to
Activity Active in job esp walking, travels freq, little time for exercise
Elimination Bowel regular q.o.d. urine 3x daily, normal stream
Meals/diet Prefers low fat diet, freq. skips breakfast
Smoking 2 packs cigarettes daily
Alcoholic beverages/drugs Heavy drinker x 15 year, stopped 2 yrs ago
Occupation Computer salesman Work Hours no set pattern 8-12 hrs/day
Hobbies Golf, reading
Marital status Divorced   Family Members 2 teenage children
Present living situation lives in 2 story home with children

INFORMATION OBTAINED FROM: client

Signature Barbara A Miller   Status RN
Date 6/11/85 Time 2:45 pm
G121 Rev. 8/84

Figure 2–5 □ Documentation of client Ted Alexander. (Courtesy of Hamilton Hospital, Trenton, NJ.)

Illustration continued on opposite page

GENERAL PHYSICAL APPEARANCE: _Well nourished white male in acute distress, c/o RLQ pain. Exam deferred until pain medication administered and effective_

SYSTEMS REVIEW

EENT: _Acuity normal c̄ corrective lens, no discharge from eyes, ears, nose. Sclera white_

Neurological: _Pupils equal and react briskly to light, hand grasps strong & equal. No history of seizures, tremors. Alert, oriented and responsive_

Pulmonary: _Breath sounds clear bilaterally. Coughs freq. Smokes to relieve tension_

Cardiovascular: _Radial, femoral and pedal pulses palpable and equal bilaterally. Pulse rapid (116) and strong BP 140/80. No neck vein distention._

Gastrointestinal: _History RLQ pain and tenderness x 2 days unrelieved by Alka seltzer/sleeping pill. Abdomen rigid, tender. 3 x 5 cm mass RLQ_

Genitourinary: _Normal male genitalia. No history pain, swelling. Does not do testicular exams. Hx of urgency and nocturia_

Reproductive: _No significant findings_

LMP/Birth Control _n/a_

Musculoskeletal: _No significant findings_

Skin: _____

TYPE OF CONDITION	LOCATION	SIZE	DESCRIPTION
(1) scar		3 cm	well healed scar "childhood injury

COMMUNICATION ABILITIES: Language _Responds appropriately to questions_
Sight _wears contact lenses/glasses_ Hearing _no problems_

EMOTIONAL STATUS: _Tense throughout interview and exam, verbalizes concerns about separation from family, management by unfamiliar physicians and job demands._

PATIENT'S UNDERSTANDING OF ILLNESS AND THERAPY: _Understands and agrees to treatment plan - gastric suction, fluid and electrolyte therapy, and surgery as described by Dr Good_

FAMILY INVOLVEMENT AND UNDERSTANDING: _Family not present. Client intends to contact children and ex-wife this pm by phone_

TEACHING NEEDS IDENTIFIED: _Preop teaching, incentive spirometry, smoking reduction or elimination_

TENTATIVE DISCHARGE PLAN: _Return to Las Vegas with the assistance of Social Service c̄ copy of discharge summary and followup by personal physician_

R.N. SIGNATURE _Barbara A. Miller RN_ DATE _6/11/85_ TIME _4:30 pm_

Figure 2–5 *Continued*

Data Collection

Many systems provide for computerized history-taking. This may be accomplished directly or indirectly. In direct systems, the client uses a computer terminal to respond to a series of questions. These histories have been demonstrated to be valid when compared with those taken indirectly and are frequently more complete and accurate (Andreoli and Musser, 1985). In indirect systems, the nurse obtains the information from the client and enters it into a bedside terminal.

Computerized systems are particularly valuable in automating physical examination. Computer terminals located at the bedside prompt the nurse to complete examinations using the body systems, head-to-toe, or functional health patterns approaches. Figure 2–6 demonstrates a sample screen used in a body systems approach.

Computers frequently provide objective data when located in technologically advanced areas, such as critical care units. Automated readings of vital signs and abnormal heart rhythms are frequently utilized by critical care nurses to provide both initial and subsequent data. "The computer can detect arrhythmias, generate alarms for vital signs ranging out of safe bound[s], store records of unusual events, provide graphic representation of vital sign trends and correlate vital signs to reveal unsuspected relationship" (Tamarisk, 1982).

Documentation

Nurses may also use computers to document the data obtained in the interview or examination. The nurse enters the data either at the bedside or in a central location. When a significant health problem is identified, the computer assists the nurse to document it accurately and completely. For example, if the nurse enters data indicating a reddened area on the client's skin, the computer will prompt for information such as location, size, and drainage. (Tamarisk, 1982). Figure 2–7 demonstrates a sample of a documented nursing assessment.

The principal advantages of computerized data collection are thoroughness and ease of recording data. The step-by-step design of the assessment process ensures that no significant areas are overlooked. Use of the computer reduces the amount of clinical time required to enter information using the traditional pen and paper format, thus improving efficiency.

The primary disadvantages of computerized client records include the expense, the time required to develop or adapt program components,

```
17WES-0301              NYUMC HOSP 4
MATRIX # 1107      HOSP# 04      03/29/85
DYNAMIC MATRIX


(N)           PHYSICAL ASSESSMENT          PG1      01
                       SKIN                          02
         *SKIN ASSESSMENT UNREMARKABLE               03
   *SKIN ASSESS'T UNCHANGED FROM PREV. NOTE          04
                                                     05

     (SKIN COLOR)        (TEMP)(MOISTURE)            06
   NORMAL      JAUNDICE    COOL  NORMAL              07
   ASHEN       PALE        HOT   DRY                 08
   DUSKY       PURPLISH    WARM  OILY                09
   CYANOTIC                      DIAPHORETIC         10
   ERYTHEMATOUS                                      11
                                      EDEMA          12
     (TEXTURE)    (TURGOR)     ANKLE                 13
     LEATHERY    ELASTIC       ARM                   14
     ROUGH       INELASTIC     HAND                  15
     SMOOTH      LOOSE         PERIORBITAL           16
     THICK       TAUT          SACRAL                17
     THIN                      PEDAL                 18
                                   *SKIN PG2         19
            *BACK    *NEXT     *ANATOMY              20
  ------------------------------------------
   RETURN                          REVIEW
  ERR        TYPE      RETRIEVE
```

```
17WES-1019              NYUMC HOSP 4
MATRIX # 1108      HOSP# 04      05/28/85
DYNAMIC MATRIX


(N)           PHYSICAL ASSESSMENT          PG2      01
                       SKIN                          02
       (NAILS)                   (HAIR)              03
   NORMAL      BRITTLE     NORMAL    THIN            04
   PALE        THIN        ALOPECIA  THICK           05
   CYANOTIC    THICK       HIRSUTE                   06
   CLUBBED     RIDGED      SCALY SCALP               07
   DYSTROPIC                                         08
   (SKIN LESION)  FRECKLE      PUSTULE               09
   ABRASION      FISSURE       PURPURA               10
   BIRTHMARK     LACERATION    RASH                  11
   BULLA         LUMP          SCALE                 12
   CALLOUS       MASS          SCAR                  13
   CRUST         MOLE          STRIAE                14
   ECCHYMOSIS    NEVI          ULCER                 15
   DECUBITUS     PETECHIAE     VESICLE               16
   EROSION       PLAQUE        WHEAL                 17
   --___           **       *DESCRIPTION             18
   SIZE--__        **       *COLOR,CONS              19
            *BACK    *NEXT     *ANATOMY              20
  ------------------------------------------------
   RETURN                          REVIEW
  ERR        TYPE      RETRIEVE
```

Figure 2–6 □ Computerized assessment screen. (Courtesy of New York University Medical Center)

```
13EAS-0217            NYUMC HOSP 4
05/28/85 12:00 NN                PAGE 001

========================================
DEMONSTRATION DAN-1          1336
4392877 85464  04/02/40  44   M
MARKS CLEMENT MD                              DEMONSTRATION DAN-1
========================================================================
                    ADMITTED  02/05/85    2:54PM
========================================================================
```

ADMITTING DIAGNOSIS:

     GI BLEED

ALLERGIES:

02/05 4:00PM
       ALLERGIES: IODINE, REACTION: RASH/HIVES

VITAL SIGNS:

       TEMP:98.8, ORAL
       RESPIRATORY RATE-24 REGULAR RHYTHM
       BP-130/90, RT ARM, LYING
       PULSE A-96
       PULSE R-96
       HT:6FT 1 IN
       WT:150 LB

PHYSICAL ASSESSMENT:

SKIN:
       SKIN COLOR NORMAL, COOL, DRY, LEATHERY TEXTURE, ELASTIC TURGOR
       NORMAL NAILS
       THIN HAIR
02/05 7:00PM
       SKIN LESION....DECUBITUS --LOCATED ON COCCYX 0.5CM. WHITE IN
       CENTER WITH NECROTIC EDGES.
NEUROLOGICAL:
02/05 4:00PM
       LEVEL OF CONSCIOUSNESS: ALERT: FOLLOWS COMMANDS: ORIENTED TO,
       PERSON, PLACE, TIME
       VERBAL RESPONSE APPROPRIATE, PT FULLY CONVERSANT
HEAD AND NECK:
       FACIAL EXPRESSION SYMMETRICAL
       SKULL: NORMOCEPHALIC
       NECK FULL ROM
RESPIRATORY:
       CHEST EXPANSION: SYMMETRICAL
       BREATH SOUNDS PRESENT ALL LUNG FIELDS.
       FINE RALES ON INSPIRATION
       NON-PRODUCTIVE COUGH
CHEST AND AXILLARY:
       CHEST&AXILLIARY ASSESS'T UNREMARKABLE
ABDOMEN:
       ABDOMEN: SYMMETRICAL

                         CONTINUED

```
========================================================================
DEMONSTRATION DAN-1                          ADMISSION NURSING NOTES
```

Figure 2–7 □ Computerized assessment: documentation. (Courtesy of New York University Medical Center)

Illustration continued on opposite page

```
05/28/85  12:00 NN              PAGE 002                        H H
                                                           HHHH
                                                           H H H
==================================                          HHHHH    H H
DEMONSTRATION DAN-1          1336                           H   H    H H
4392877 85464  04/02/40  44   M                          ===================
MARKS CLEMENT MD                                         DEMONSTRATION DAN-1
==========================================================================
              ADMITTED  02/05/85    2:54PM
==========================================================================
     BOWEL SOUNDS ABSENT
MUSCULO-SKELETAL:
     MUS/SKEL ASSESS'T UNREMARKABLE
```

PATTERN OF DAILY LIVING:

```
COMMUNICATIONS:
     PT HAS VALUABLES/PROPERTY, YES
     ORIENTED TO UNIT/FLOOR ROUTINE
SENSORY IMPAIRMENT:
     PT WEARS GLASSES
ACTIVITY:
     ACTIVITY: AD LIB, WALKS 4 BLOCKS
     BATHING, INDEPEND'T
     MOUTH CARE, INDEPEND'T
     DRESSING, INDEPEND'T
DIET:
     DIET: NO ADDED SALT.
     FREQUENT INDIGESTION.
     WT LOSS X3WKS 20LBS
     APPETITE POOR
     PT HAS CAPS ON TEETH
SLEEP:
     SLEEP PATTERN, NO DIFFICULTY
     USES NIGHTLIGHT
     USES 3 PILLOWS
ELIMINATION:
     BLADDER PATTERN NOCTURIA/X1
     BOWEL PATTERN REGULAR
HEALTH HABITS:
     ALCOHOL: DENIES
     SMOKING: DENIES
     KNOWN INFECTION AT ADMISSION- NO
```

PROJECTED DISCHARGE:

```
     PROJECTED DISCHARGE TO: HOME, WITH SIGNIF OTHER
     DISCHARGE TEACHING NEEDS: DIET
     DISCHARGE TEACHING NEEDS: MEDICATION
     DISCHARGE TEACHING NEEDS: DISEASE PROCESS


               KELLY,JANET B.     RN   JBKA


               LASTPAGE
```

```
==========================================================================
DEMONSTRATION DAN-1                            ADMISSION NURSING NOTES
- k-
```

Figure 2–7 *Continued*

and the training required prior to use. Additionally, some object to the restrictions imposed by standardized screens, formats, and limited vocabulary (Gluck, 1980).

SUMMARY

The assessment phase of the nursing process consists of the accumulation and documentation of information about a client. Data collection involves interviewing, observation, and physical examination and concludes with documentation of the information obtained in the client's medical record. Assessment involves interaction between the nurse and the client and requires a broad knowledge base as well as specific interpersonal and technical skills. Assessment is a continuous activity that begins at the time of admission and continues during each client contact. It forms the foundation for subsequent phases of the nursing process—diagnosis, planning, implementation, and evaluation.

References

American Nurses' Association: Standards of Nursing Practice. Kansas City, MO: American Nurses' Association, 1973.
American Nurses' Association: Nursing: A Social Policy Statement. Kansas City, MO: American Nurses' Association, 1980.
Andreoli K and Musser L: Computers in nursing care: the state of the art. Nursing Outlook 33(1):16–25, 1985.
Bellack J and Bamford P: Nursing Assessment. California: Wadsworth, Inc., 1984.
Gluck J: The computerized medical record system: meeting the challenge for nursing. In Zielstorff R: Computers in Nursing. Rockville, Maryland: Aspen, 1980.
Tamarisk NK: The computer as a clinical tool. Nursing Management 13(8):46–49, 1982.

Bibliography

Bates B: A Guide to Physical Examination. 2nd ed. Philadelphia: JB Lippincott, 1979.
Carnevali D: Nursing Care Planning. 3rd ed. Philadelphia: JB Lippincott, 1983.
Carpenito LJ: Nursing Diagnosis—Application to Clinical Practice. Philadelphia: JB Lippincott, 1983.
Eggland ET: Charting: how and why to document your care daily and fully. Nursing '80 10:38–43, 1980.
Fiesta J: The Law and Liability—A Guide for Nurses. New York: John Wiley & Sons, 1983.
Gordon M: Nursing Diagnosis: Process and Application. New York: McGraw-Hill, 1982.
Grobe S: Computer Primer and Resources Guide for Nurses. Philadelphia: JB Lippincott, 1984.
Hemelt MD and Mackert ME: Dynamics of Law in Nursing and Health Care. 2nd ed. Reston, Virginia: Reston, 1982.
Kerr AH: Nurses' notes—that's where the goodies are. Nursing '75 5:34–41, 1975.
Kozier B and Erb G: Fundamentals of Nursing. 2nd ed. Menlo Park, California: Addison-Wesley, 1983.

Luckmann J and Sorensen K: Medical Surgical Nursing: A Psychophysiologic Approach. 2nd ed. Philadelphia: WB Saunders, 1980.

Malasanos L: Health Assessment. 2nd ed. St. Louis: CV Mosby, 1981.

Marriner A: The Nursing Process: A Scientific Approach to Nursing Care. 3rd ed. St. Louis: CV Mosby, 1982.

Mitchell PH: Concepts Basic to Nursing. 2nd ed. New York: McGraw-Hill, 1977.

Moritz DA: Nursing histories—a guide, yes, a form, no! Oncology Nursing Forum 6:18–19, 1979.

Murray M: Fundamentals of Nursing. 2nd ed. Englewood Cliffs, New Jersey: Prentice-Hall, Inc., 1980.

Phipps WJ, Long BC, and Woods NF (eds): Medical-Surgical Nursing: Concepts and Clinical Practice. 2nd ed. St. Louis: CV Mosby, 1983.

Powel NM: Designing and developing a computerized hospital information system. Nursing Management 13(8):40–45, 1982.

Reaves DM and Underly NK: Computerization of nursing. Nursing Management 13(8):50–53, 1982.

Robinson J (ed): Documenting Patient Care Responsibly. Horsham, Pennsylvania: Intermed Communications, 1978.

Romano C, McCormack KA, and McNeely LD: Nursing documentation: a model for a computerized data base. Advances in Nursing Science 4(2):43–56, 1982.

Smith VM and Bass TA: Communication for Health Professionals. Philadelphia: JB Lippincott, 1979.

Thomas E: How to take a meaningful history. Nursing '77 7:22–30, 1977.

Yura H and Walsh MB: The Nursing Process. 4th ed. New York: Appleton-Century-Crofts, 1983.

Nursing Diagnosis

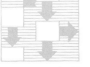

STEPS IN THE DIAGNOSTIC PROCESS

There are four steps involved in the diagnostic phase of the nursing process—data processing, formulation of the nursing diagnosis, verification, and documentation. The data processing component involves classification, interpretation, and validation. This chapter will explore the data processing component as well as the concept of nursing diagnosis. Chapter 4 will describe how to write, verify, and document a nursing diagnosis.

Data Processing

The information collected by the nurse about an individual client is vital to the development of the nursing diagnosis and subsequent nursing care planning. Before the planning phase can occur, data must be processed—classified, interpreted, and validated. Although data processing will be examined as the first phase of diagnosis, it is not so specifically isolated. These activities are dynamic rather than static and occur continuously throughout the nursing process.

Classification

During the assessment of a client, the nurse accumulates a massive volume of data. The nurse may find it extremely difficult to manage this volume in total. The classification process results in the development of more manageable categories of information. It also stimulates discrimination between data. This allows the nurse to focus on data that are pertinent to the client's needs.

Classification involves the sorting of information into specific categories. Frequently this process is facilitated by the format of the assessment tool.

Examples

Data	Classification
Appendectomy three years ago	Past medical history
Sleeps during the day	Sleep/rest pattern
Full range of motion	Motor ability
Colostomy	Gastrointestinal system
Mother died of cancer	Family history
Laxatives every other day	Bowel elimination pattern
Church elder	Spiritual history
Vomiting for three days	History of present illness
Sacral redness	Integumentary

Categorization also assists the nurse to begin to identify and collect missing data during the interview and physical examination.

Example. Joan Evans is a 45 year old woman admitted for cholecystitis. During the interview she indicates that her mother died of cancer of the breast (family history) and that she had a breast biopsy two years ago (past medical history).

Classification of this information reveals a missing component—current status of breast disease. Therefore, the nurse might (1) question the client regarding the outcome of the biopsy and frequency of self-breast examination, (2) pay particular attention to palpation for breast masses during the physical examination, and (3) assess the client's emotional response to this potential health problem.

Interpretation

The second step in the processing of data is interpretation. This involves the identification of significant data, comparison with standards or norms, and recognition of patterns or trends. The use of cues and inferences is particularly valuable. A cue is a piece of information obtained about an individual client through the use of the five senses. It is the nurse's perception of what exists based on subjective and objective data obtained from the client and other secondary sources. Each bit of information obtained during the assessment phase could be considered a cue.

Examples

Temperature 102° F
Grimacing
6 ft, 275 lb
White blood count 24,000/mm³ (normal 5000 to 9000/mm³)

Inferencing is the assignment of meaning to a cue or group of cues. In the examples identified above, the nurse might make the following judgments based on the cues.

Cues	Inference
Temperature 102° F	Elevated temperature
Grimacing	Possible pain, anxiety
6 ft, 275 lb	Obesity
White blood count 24,000/mm³	Probable infection

The use of a group of cues to make an inference increases the potential for accurate judgments. In the case of the client with a temperature elevation, note that two different inferences could be identified based on additional cues.

Cues	Inference
Temperature 102° F White blood count 24,000/mm³ Reddened incision Purulent drainage	Incision is infected

Cues	Inference
Temperature 102° F Decreased skin turgor Dry tongue Urine output 200 ml in 8 hr	Client is dehydrated

The nurse uses a theoretical knowledge base, experience, and data gathered about the client to make correct inferences. Some inferences are very clear, based on a clinical knowledge. For example, the presence of chest pain, blood work that indicates elevated cardiac enzymes, and an injury pattern on an EKG imply the presence of cardiac disease, specifically a myocardial infarction. Other data may provide fewer concrete cues and require more interpretation. The client with clenched fists and rigid body posture who is crying may be angry, frightened, or experiencing pain. Two individual nurses may interpret these cues very differently based on their knowledge, experience, and information about the client.

Inductive Reasoning. The nurse may use inductive or deductive reasoning to interpret data. Inductive reasoning begins with a set of facts and results in a conclusion.

Example. James McKany is an 84 year old client admitted with a fractured hip. He is thin, has dry skin, and is on bedrest with traction.

The nurse recognizes that based on his age, body build, skin condition, and immobility (set of facts) this client is at rest for altered skin integrity (conclusion).

Example. Nancy Angelis is an experienced postpartum nurse who has worked with hundreds of mothers who have breast fed their infants. She has observed anxiety in a number of first-time nursing mothers.

In this situation, Nancy concludes that most first-time nursing mothers experience anxiety about their ability to breast-feed. This is inductive inferencing because the nurse's generalization (conclusion) about breast-feeding mothers is based on a group of observations (set of facts). It moves from the particular to the general.

Deductive Reasoning. Deductive reasoning on the other hand begins with a major premise or generalization and proceeds to the specifics.

Example. Joan Granberry is a nurse on a 24 bed surgical unit. Her clinical knowledge indicates that pain is a common phenomenon in the post-op client. Based on this knowledge, she observes her client for indications of tense body posture, restlessness, moaning, limited range of motion, rapid pulse, and elevated blood pressure.

This is deductive inferencing because the nurse uses generalized knowledge about postoperative clients to anticipate the pain response in a specific situation.

Example. Mr. Devine is an admitted alcoholic currently under treatment for pancreatitis. On admission, Mr. Devine reveals that he had his last drink that morning. The nurse recognizes that interruption of his drinking pattern will result in alcohol withdrawal symptoms (delirium tremens) within 72 hours of admission unless he receives sedation. The nurse discusses this problem with the physician, who subsequently orders sedation.

3–1 TEST YOURSELF

IDENTIFICATION OF INFERENCES

Read the cues/clusters in column I and identify possible inferences in column II.

Cue/Cluster   **Inference**

1. Blood pressure 90/50 mm Hg
   (normally 120/70)
2. Bright red vaginal bleeding
   (one pad in six hours)
3. Urine glucose 2% (normal = 0)
4. Dilated pupils in an alert, oriented client
5. Height 5 ft, 1 in; weight 220 lb; pendulous abdomen
6. Blood pressure 190/104 mm Hg; client states "I wasn't supposed to eat salt."
7. Whimpering one year old child; restlessness; pulling left ear
8. Insomnia; heart rate 110 beats/min; irritability; verbalizes feelings of "nervousness"
9. History of accidents; unsteady gait; impaired vision
10. Newly diagnosed diabetic; states "I've never tested urine before;" inaccurate test results

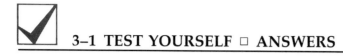

3–1 TEST YOURSELF □ ANSWERS

Read the cues/clusters in column I and identify possible inferences in column II.

Cues/Cluster	Inference
1. Blood pressure 90/50 mm Hg (normally 120/70)	Abnormally low for client
2. Bright red vaginal bleeding (one pad in six hours)	Menstruation
3. Urine glucose 2% (normal = 0)	Abnormal glucose level
4. Dilated pupils in an alert, oriented client	Medication effects
5. Height 5 ft, 1 in; weight 220 lb; pendulous abdomen	Obesity
6. Blood pressure 190/104 mm Hg; client states "I wasn't supposed to eat salt."	Abnormally elevated blood pressure
7. Whimpering one year old child; restlessness; pulling left ear	Pain in left ear
8. Insomnia; heart rate 110 beats/min; irritability; verbalizes feelings of "nervousness"	Anxiety
9. History of accidents; unsteady gait; impaired vision	Potential for injury
10. Newly diagnosed diabetic; states "I've never tested urine before;" inaccurate test results	Lack of knowledge about urine testing

Validation

The final step in data processing is validation. In this phase the nurse attempts to verify the accuracy of data interpretation. This may be accomplished by direct interaction with the client or significant other(s), consultation with other health care professionals, or comparison of data with an authoritative reference.

Validation with the Client/Family. Ideally, the nurse should validate findings with the client. This is generally accomplished through the use of reflective statements.

Example. Sally Furey is a 26 year old client admitted for an elective cesarean section. During the assessment interview the nurse notices that

Sally is easily distracted, paces intermittently while wringing her hands, and speaks very rapidly. These cues could lead the nurse to infer that this client is anxious about the scheduled surgery.

Nurse: You seem anxious Mrs. Furey.
Client: Yes, I am upset.
Nurse: Upset?
Client: I'm really worried about my two year old. She had a high fever so my husband took her to the doctor. He hasn't called me yet to tell me what the doctor found. I'm so afraid that she had pneumonia.

In this situation, the nurse validated the presence of anxiety in the client. The use of a reflected statement negated the nurse's interpretation of the source of the client's anxiety. The nurse was able to identify that Mrs. Furey's concern was focused on the welfare of her child. Therefore, nursing interventions would be directed toward assisting the client to resolve those fears.

Occasionally, it may not be desirable or possible to validate interpretations with the client directly. In some situations, the nurse may determine that it is not appropriate to validate interpretations verbally with the client.

Example. Susan Dugan, a nurse in the prenatal clinic, is interviewing Kim Percell, who is six months pregnant with her first child. The nurse notices that Kim has edema in her hands and feet and that she has gained ten pounds since her visit last month.

In this instance, the nurse suspects toxemia of pregnancy and chooses to validate her interpretation by measuring the client's blood pressure and testing her urine for albumin. The nurse avoids sharing her concerns with Susan until she confirms her findings with the physician.

Example. The nurse admitting a comatose client, James Flemming, notices a small healed scar approximately 2½ in long just below the left clavicle. There is also a small bulge under the client's skin. Based on knowledge and past experience, the nurse interprets these findings as indicating the presence of a cardiac pacemaker.

In this situation, the client is unable to confirm the nurse's perception. Therefore Mr. Flemming's daughter might be interviewed for confirmation.

Nurse: I noticed that your father has a small scar on his chest.
Daughter: Yes he had a pacemaker put in six months ago after his heart attack. He has it checked every month, and it's been working fine.

The daughter has validated the presence of the pacemaker and in that process has provided additional important data regarding the client's past medical history as well as his compliance with follow-up management.

Validation with Other Professionals. Another method of validation is collaboration with other health professionals. In the case of James Flemming described previously, the nurse was able to verify the presence of a cardiac pacemaker through discussion with the client's family. In the absence of the daughter, however, the nurse might have contacted the attending physician, obtained the client's old chart from medical records, or consulted with nurses in the coronary care unit.

Example. Stephanie French is a 48 year old client with a diagnosis of metastatic cancer of the colon. She is four days post-op after surgery for a permanent ileostomy. Based on her observations of the client, the nurse identifies cues indicating that the client is denying her diagnosis. Subsequent discussion with the client's physician and the stomal therapist verifies the nurse's impression.

Validation with Reference Sources. The nurse may also use reference sources to substantiate interpretations.

Example. Jenny is an eight month old admitted to a same day surgery unit for a tear duct probing. The nurse notices that the child does not turn over independently, sit unaided, or hold her bottle.

In this situation the nurse might use a pediatric reference source to verify initial perceptions that Jenny is not at an appropriate developmental level for her age. Reference sources might include texts, journals, or developmental charts.

Validation is an important component of the diagnostic process. The approaches just described facilitate verification of the accuracy and completeness of the nurse's interpretations. Validation assists the nurse to recognize errors, isolate discrepancies, and identify the need for additional information. This phase in the processing of data forms the bridge between assessment and formulation of nursing diagnoses.

ERRORS IN THE DIAGNOSTIC PROCESS

Introduction

Up to this point, the text has presented information on data collection, organization, interpretation, and validation. These are the components necessary for the diagnostic process. The nurse gathers data, identifies cues, makes inferences about the health status of the client, and validates these perceptions with the client. The outcome of this process is a label—the *nursing diagnosis*. If any of these steps are carried out incorrectly or incompletely, the label may be inaccurate.

There are three major sources of error in the diagnostic process. They are (1) inaccurate or incomplete data collection, (2) inaccurate interpretation of data, and (3) lack of clinical knowledge.

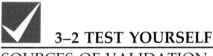

3–2 TEST YOURSELF

SOURCES OF VALIDATION

Identify methods of validation that might be used by the nurse in the situations described below.

Validation
A. Directly with client/family
B. Collaboration with health care professionals
C. Reference sources

Situation
1. Nathan Ram is seen in the outpatient clinic on a well baby visit. He is 18 months old and weighs 18 pounds. His mother asks, "Is he underweight?" How can this be determined?
2. A 17 year old teenager is brought into the Emergency Department complaining of stomach pain. Shortly after he is placed on a stretcher, he vomits brown liquid. The nurse realizes that the vomitus could be old blood but knows that certain liquids, such as coffee or hot chocolate, can resemble old blood. What should the nurse do to pursue this?
3. Jason Mebain, a 19 year old college sophomore, is seen at the university student health center because of his claims that voices are telling him to kill his English professor. The nurse practitioner interviews Jason to obtain more information about his thought processes. During the discussion, Jason indicates that Dr. Mimi Johnson saw him three weeks ago when he had these same feelings. What would be the appropriate next step?

✔️ **3–2   TEST YOURSELF □ ANSWERS**

1. C—Consult a growth chart (reference source).
2. A—Ask the client or family about any intake of coffee or hot chocolate.
3. B—Contact Dr. Johnson.

Inaccurate or Incomplete Data Collection

The nurse's ability to formulate nursing diagnoses is dependent on an accurate and complete data base. Several factors may interfere with the collection of data. These may include any of the following interviewing difficulties.

1. Either the client or the nurse may have a language barrier that makes communication difficult. Even when the nurse and client speak the same language, either may use slang or jargon that confuses the other. The client's cultural background might involve the use of expressions that are totally foreign to the nurse. In turn, the nurse might talk in technical jargon or use a vocabulary that is above the client's level of understanding.

The lack of ability to communicate clearly leads to a data base that may be deficient. Important pieces of information may not be shared or understood. Communication problems can be minimized when both client and nurse make an effort to express themselves with easily understandable words. Misunderstandings may be detected by watching facial expressions for evidence of comprehension or by asking the client to repeat something in his or her own words.

2. Biased questions, as described in Chapter 2, tend to intimidate clients and frequently affect communication. When clients give the responses they believe are expected, the data obtained may be inaccurate. Biased questions should be avoided whenever possible.

3. Withholding of information may lead to an inaccurate and incomplete data base. Clients may fail to share information out of anxiety, embarrassment, suspicion, or lack of awareness of its importance. When obtaining information, the nurse should make every effort to put the client at ease, explain why the questions are being asked, and explore all pertinent areas.

4. Distractions can interfere with the concentration required to collect data. Distracting factors can include interruptions, a noisy, nonprivate environment, or thoughts that are preoccupying the nurse or client.

The nurse who is rushed or distracted may not listen carefully to the information provided. This can lead to an incomplete data base when a significant piece of information is overlooked.

Example. When Lester Goldstein was admitted with emphysema, he said he had no family. The nurse, who was in a hurry, did not pursue this by asking him if he had friends who would be visiting him. When Lester became progressively more depressed as his hospitalization continued, the nurses assumed that his depression was related to being chronically ill. However, one astute nurse encouraged Lester to talk. He revealed that he was upset because no one had visited him. The nurses then realized that he was withdrawn because of loneliness. The nurse who admitted him might have anticipated this problem if inquiries had been made about his support system.

Example. When Tommy, age two, was admitted with pneumonia, the nurse, Jackie, was just about to go off duty. Jackie did a quick assessment, including checking his vital signs and weight. Tommy's general appearance was pathetic. He was dirty, undernourished, and withdrawn. Jackie wondered, "Could this be an abused child?" But when she did not see any bruises or lesions on his face or arms, she wrote "skin intact without lesions" on the assessment sheet.

The next day Jackie learned that Tommy had cigarette burns on his back and buttocks. Thanks in part to the complete assessment of Ron, the night nurse, Tommy's home situation was investigated. Being in a hurry is no excuse for doing an incomplete assessment, and not noticing lesions on a client's face or arms does not justify writing "skin intact" on the assessment sheet ("Confidentially," 1983b).

In this case the nurse's failure to do a thorough assessment led to an incomplete data base. This could have been avoided if the nurse had taken the few extra minutes required to do a complete examination.

At times, certain aspects of the client's behavior can be distracting. For example, the client may wander from the subject being discussed, making it difficult for the nurse to gather the information. In the case below, the nurse allowed the conversation to be directed away from the client's hypertension, which was the reason for the client's visit to the clinic.

Example

Client:	Oh yes, I've had high blood pressure for years. I stopped watching my diet because it is too much trouble. I don't cook much since I live alone. I used to live with my sister, but she moved to Florida. She just loves it there.
Nurse:	Where is she living in Florida?
Client:	She lives in Orlando. The city is growing so fast because of the climate and the attractions. Now, that's a wonderful place. Have you ever been there?
Nurse:	Yes.
Client:	What I like best about it is the weather. I could spend months there. It is nicer than other places where I've gone. Of course, I enjoy the Houston area too. There's a darling hotel there right near the water where I've stayed four times. . . .

Clearly the nurse has lost control of the interview process and has not investigated the problem of the client's nonadherence to the diet.

Inaccurate Interpretation of Data

Two different types of errors may lead to inaccurate processing of data: (1) using only one cue or observation to reach premature inferences, and (2) allowing personal prejudices or biases to influence the processing of data.

Premature Interpretation of Data

A common type of error is the development of a diagnosis before all the important information is collected or considered. Problems can occur when only one observation is used to create a diagnosis. The nurse should rely on identification of a pattern of behavior rather than make judgments based on only one episode. This type of error occurs in the following situation.

Example. Anne Weaver puts on her call light at 4 P.M. while she is talking on the phone. The 3–11 nurse who answers her light is not familiar with

Anne's pattern of needing pain medication every three hours for arthritis. When the nurse enters the room, Anne is laughing at something that is being said on the phone. "Oh nurse," she says, "could you bring me my pain medication?" The nurse walks away thinking "How much pain could she be in if she can laugh like that?" When the nurse checks Anne's medication record, it becomes clear that Anne's request for medication represents a pattern of behavior. The telephone conversation has temporarily distracted the client's responses to the pain. The established pattern of behavior is more valid than the nurse's single observation of the client laughing.

Sometimes a nurse reaches a conclusion based on just one cue rather than investigating further. Therefore, the interpretation of the data and the resulting diagnosis may be faulty, as is true in the following case.

Example. Regina Townsend, a home care nurse, was visiting Mr. Falk at home. Mr. Falk had been discharged from the hospital with a Foley catheter. When Mrs. Falk said that urine was leaking around the catheter, Regina decided that the 5 cc balloon probably wasn't inflated enough to hold the catheter securely in place. She instilled more sterile water into the balloon.

The next day Mrs. Falk called, quite upset, saying that the urine leakage was worse and Mr. Falk was in great discomfort. When Regina visited him that day, she discovered that the catheter had dislodged from Mr. Falk's bladder. The balloon was probably in his urethra. After Regina replaced the catheter, Mr. Falk became comfortable, and the catheter stopped leaking ("Confidentially," 1983b).

Regina took one cue—a leaking catheter—and came to the wrong conclusion because she failed to gather more data before taking action. Her misinterpretation of the cue resulted in additional discomfort for Mr. Falk.

Another type of error is jumping to inaccurate conclusions using the medical diagnosis as a cue. The nurse who expects the diabetic client to behave in specific ways because of the diagnosis may be unable to recognize the individuality of the client's needs. A series of nursing diagnoses may be developed that have no bearing on the client's pressing problems. To maintain a low rate of diagnostic error, the nurse must take the time to validate interpretations of the client's problems.

Personal Prejudices

Personal prejudices and lack of awareness of cultural practices or beliefs can influence a nurse's interpretation of a client's problems. Sometimes the behavior of a client or family can become so annoying that the nurse is tempted to ignore important cues. Consider what could have happened in this situation.

Example. Mr. Allen was recovering well from gallbladder surgery, but his family hovered around as if he were at death's door. Although Mr. Allen himself never complained, his wife and two daughters had a hundred trivial requests. And they wanted everything done pronto.

One evening Mrs. Allen excitedly demanded that the nurse check Mr. Allen, who had pain in his left knee. The nurse thought "what next?" as she went into Mr. Allen's room, fully expecting another false alarm. To her surprise, she was unable to find a pulse in Mr. Allen's leg. He was rushed to surgery for removal of a blood clot. The nurse felt guilty because she had been so sure that Mrs. Allen was just overreacting ("Confidentially," 1983a).

The nurse must be in touch with personal values and biases, recognize how these influence perceptions, and attempt to overcome prejudices. When presented with unfamiliar cultural practices or beliefs, the nurse should seek out resources to assist in improving understanding of the client's responses. This will enhance the ability to interpret cues correctly.

Lack of Clinical Knowledge or Experience

Lack of clinical knowledge or experience may affect the collection and interpretation of data. It may result in critical data's not being collected or in incorrect clustering or interpretation of cues.

The inexperienced nurse may simply overlook important assessment data because of inadequate clinical knowledge. For example, the new graduate may fail to recognize that an elderly client with sacral edema is at risk for alterations in skin integrity. Or the nurse may focus so much attention on one aspect of care that a whole set of cues is ignored.

Example. Dot Battershell's first job was with a community health agency in a poor urban area. One of her first clients was a diabetic who needed instructions on planning low cost, nutritious meals. Before Dot's 30 day performance evaluation, she asked her supervisor if she would accompany Dot to the client's home to show her the progress she'd made.

The supervisor seemed impressed until she asked the client to remove her shoes and thick stockings. To Dot's dismay, the client's legs and feet were encrusted with dirt. For the next half hour, Dot bathed the client's legs and feet while her supervisor explained the importance of foot care for diabetics. Dot learned an important lesson: never get so involved with one aspect of nursing care that you overlook something equally important ("Confidentially," 1984).

Example. An 80 year old woman who had been in the hospital for ten days fell after getting out of bed at midnight to go to the bathroom. The court held the hospital liable for the nurse's negligence. The woman had received flurazepam (Dalmane) about an hour before. Although the bedrails at her head were elevated, those by her legs were down.

The manufacturer of Dalmane warns that dizziness, drowsiness, lightheadedness, staggering, ataxia, and falling have occurred with its use, particularly in elderly or debilitated persons, so the nurse should have anticipated the risk to the patient (Cushing, 1985).

If the nurse had recognized the client's potential for falling, preventive measures could have been taken. In this situation, the nurse's lack of clinical knowledge and failure to put up the siderails led to injury to the client.

Lack of knowledge of critical signs or symptoms will result in errors in clustering or interpreting data. The nurse may incorrectly identify the problem or its cause and therefore initiate inappropriate interventions.

Example. Bob Williams learned in a report that Mr. Gray, age 82, had been diagnosed as diabetic and hyperglycemic. The nurses said he was also confused, so they had restrained him. When Bob entered the room, Mr. Gray was thrashing about, talking loudly and incoherently. Bob checked his blood pressure and blood glucose level. Both were normal.

Assuming that Mr. Gray's confusion was due to his age and unfamiliar surroundings, Bob called his physician and asked if he could order sedation. The physician said he wanted to check Mr. Gray first. Ten minutes later, when the physician and Bob entered Mr. Gray's room, they found him unresponsive. They began cardiopulmonary resuscitation (CPR), and he was successfully resuscitated.

Mr. Gray's confusion was actually caused by hypoxia from an irregular heart beat. If Bob had checked the chart, he would have seen that Mr. Gray had a history of irregular heart beats. The nurse learned that it is better to prevent such life-threatening situations by avoiding the temptation to jump to conclusions ("Confidentially," 1985).

If Mr. Gray's physician had granted Bob's request for sedation, the client's condition would have been further compromised. The nurse who lacks adequate clinical knowledge or experience can compensate for these deficits by seeking information and guidance from appropriate resources. The general rule—"When in doubt, ask"—holds true when the nurse is faced with the task of interpreting difficult data.

NURSING DIAGNOSIS

Before attempting to develop diagnostic statements, it may be helpful to define and explore the evolution of the concept of *nursing diagnosis.*

Definitions of Nursing Diagnosis

A diagnosis is essentially a statement that identifies the existence of an undesirable state. This definition applies whether the diagnostician is a health care worker, lawyer, electrician, or mechanic. The subject matter of the diagnoses consists of those areas in which the diagnostician possesses a level of expertise. Lawyers write diagnoses pertaining to the elements of law, physicians diagnose disease states, and electricians identify electrical system malfunctions.

Nurses, by virtue of their nurse practice acts, are responsible for diagnosing and treating human responses to health problems. Nursing diagnosis primarily involves examining those areas that have been identified as independent nursing functions, which can be ordered independently without collaboration with physicians or other health care professionals. These functions may include (1) preventive approaches, such as education, changes of position, or observation for problems, or (2) corrective approaches, such as forcing fluids and treatments. This focus on independent nursing actions not only avoids duplication and overlap with other disciplines but also continues the definition and validation of the elements of nursing practice.

There have been several definitions of nursing diagnosis. A few of these are listed below.

- □ A nursing diagnosis is a statement of a patient problem that is arrived at by making inferences from the collected data. The problem is one that can be alleviated by nursing (Mundinger and Jauron, 1975).
- □ Nursing diagnoses, or clinical diagnoses made by professional nurses, describe actual or potential health problems that nurses, by virtue of their education and experience, are capable and licensed to treat (Gordon, 1976).
- □ The American Nurses' Association emphasizes the importance of nursing diagnoses in its definition of nursing: nursing is the diagnosis and treatment of human responses to actual or potential health problems (ANA, 1980).

For the purposes of this discussion, a commonly accepted definition will be used—a nursing diagnosis is a label for a patient condition (response to health or illness) that nurses are able and legally responsible to treat (Moritz, 1982).

Regardless of which definition is used, the experts agree that a nursing diagnosis includes certain essential features, which are identified in Table 3–1.

TABLE 3–1 □ A NURSING DIAGNOSIS . . .

□ is a statement of a client problem
□ refers to a health state or a potential health problem
□ is a conclusion resulting from identification of a pattern or cluster of signs and symptoms
□ is based on subjective and objective data that can be confirmed
□ is a statement of nursing judgment
□ refers to a condition that nurses are licensed to treat
□ refers to physical, psychological, sociocultural, and spiritual conditions
□ is a short, concise statement
□ is a two-part statement that includes the etiology when known
□ refers to conditions that can be treated independently by a nurse
□ should be validated with the client whenever possible

Adapted from Shoemaker J: Essential features of a nursing diagnosis. In McLane M, McFarland K, and Kim M (eds): Classification of Nursing Diagnoses: Proceedings of the Fifth National Conference. St. Louis: CV Mosby, 1984, 107–108.

Historical Evolution of Nursing Diagnosis

Chapter 1 described the historical evolution of the nursing process. The term *nursing diagnosis* was first used in the 1950s. In 1960, Faye Abdellah introduced a classification system for identifying 21 clinical problems. This system was used in the curriculum of nursing schools to assist students to identify client problems.

In the 1970s, several nursing leaders recognized the need to develop terminology to describe the health problems diagnosed and treated by nurses. In 1973, the First National Conference on the Classification of Nursing Diagnoses was held at the St. Louis University School of Nursing. The group began to formulate nursing diagnoses and published a tentative list. Since then, the group has continued to meet to develop and refine nursing diagnoses.

The American Nurses' Association endorsed and legitimized the use of the term *nursing diagnosis* in 1973 by publishing standards of nursing practice. Standard II states "Nursing diagnoses are derived from the data of the health status of the client." Subsequently, several states began incorporating the term into their nurse practice acts. This provided nurses with a legal right as well as an obligation to make nursing diagnoses. At this time nursing diagnosis was viewed as an outcome or label that resulted from the diagnostic process. The development of the nursing diagnosis became the second step of the five step nursing process.

Throughout the 1970s and into the 1980s, a great deal of nursing literature explained the concepts of nursing diagnosis and nursing process. The acceptance and usage of nursing diagnoses have resulted from the sharing of ideas and the education of student and graduate nurses.

The Controversy Surrounding Nursing Diagnoses

The concept of the nursing diagnosis has created more controversy than any other aspect of the nursing process. Its introduction in the 1970s was accompanied by numerous articles supporting its use and citing its advantages. However, many of the practicing nurses who were asked to write nursing diagnoses greeted the idea with resistance. It is important to look at this issue from both sides by examining the benefits of nursing diagnoses as well as the reasons for resistance by nurses.

Objections to Nursing Diagnoses

1. Writing a nursing diagnosis requires time to gather data and validate the diagnosis. Patients in hospitals are now sicker and are going home sooner than in the past. Nurses in acute care settings have less time than ever to identify, diagnose, and treat nursing problems.

Response. This is a legitimate concern that will increase in importance as cost containment efforts create even shorter lengths of hospital stay. However, the nursing diagnosis is the pivotal part of the nursing process. It helps to determine goals and interventions. The effectiveness of the interventions hinges on its accuracy. Therefore, the time taken to formulate nursing diagnoses and to plan care results in increased efficiency, better utilization of time for all nursing staff, and the provision of appropriate nursing care.

2. Many nurses in acute care settings still organize their care directly around the medical diagnosis. Clients and physicians reinforce this pattern by expecting that the nurse will spend the majority of time following

medical orders. Nurses are rewarded for completion of tasks, not for writing nursing diagnoses.

Response. Nurses who plan care exclusively around the medical diagnoses are limited when the diagnosis is incomplete or absent. Further, the medical diagnosis is narrow, in that it focuses only on pathology, whereas nursing is involved with the psychological, social, spiritual, and physiological responses of the client. Nursing diagnoses help to clarify the role of the nurse by identifying the scope of nursing practice. By being able to define nursing's unique contribution to health care, two goals are accomplished: (1) nursing diagnoses form the basis of nursing education and create a sense of direction for research, and (2) nursing diagnoses are useful in explaining nursing to the public, legislators, administrators, third party payers, and professional colleagues.

Nursing practice is no longer limited to carrying out medical orders. As defined by the ANA standards and nurse practice acts, nurses are held accountable for making accurate nursing diagnoses.

3. Many nurses, when learning to write nursing diagnoses, are afraid that they will make an error that will open them to ridicule or criticism. They feel it is better not to take the risk than to be wrong.

Response. Most peers are supportive and willing to help each other learn. As nurses gain experience in formulating nursing diagnoses, the process becomes easier. Although it involves a certain amount of risk to document a judgment that may be perceived by others as being incorrect, risk-taking is part of being a professional.

4. Nursing diagnoses limit nursing practice by forcing adherence to a list of clumsy labels.

Response. The process of formulating a nursing diagnosis requires theoretical knowledge, analytical thinking, and a willingness to keep an open mind to explore all possibilities. There will be cases in which there are no accepted nursing diagnoses that fit the pattern the nurse has identified. These cases form the basis for development of new diagnostic labels.

Since one of the purposes of nursing diagnosis is to communicate clearly in nursing's professional language, any diagnostic statement should be easily understood. Since the terminology is in an early stage, it tends to be clumsy or wordy. The expectation is that this will change. After all, it took hundreds of years to perfect medical diagnoses.

The National Conference System

There are several ways to state nursing diagnoses. The methods of organizing them are called classification systems. The most commonly used system is the National Conference System. A survey of 74 National League for Nursing (NLN) accredited baccalaureate and higher degree programs found that 81.5 per cent of the programs taught the use of the National Conference System (Gaines and McFarland, 1984).

Development

The National Conference System grew out of the First National Conference held in 1973. Conferences to discuss nursing diagnoses have been held approximately every two years since then.

The participants at the First National Conference were assigned to ten groups. Each group was asked to consider a human system and to develop possible diagnostic labels. At the first three national conferences, the small groups generated labels, and the conference as a whole determined whether a given label would be published on the list of accepted diagnostic labels. At the Fourth and Fifth Conferences, small groups made recommendations, but the participants had no role in decision-making. This role became the responsibility of the Task Force, a group of 36 nursing leaders from all regions of the country, representing a variety of practice areas. The Task Force was established in 1973 and changed its name to the North American Nursing Diagnosis Association (NANDA) in 1982.

NANDA's responsibilities include

□ Reviewing and editing the recommendations of the conference's small groups;
□ Sharing information and providing education about nursing diagnoses at the state, regional, and national levels;
□ Promoting research and development activities;
□ Planning for the national conferences.

A Nursing Diagnosis Newsletter, published by the Clearinghouse for Nursing Diagnoses at St. Louis University, assists NANDA in sharing information about nursing diagnoses. The newsletter encourages nurses to ask questions, exchange views, submit articles, and share experiences on the implementation of diagnoses in practice, research, and education. Nurses may subscribe to the newsletter by contacting

North American Nursing Diagnosis Association
St. Louis University Department of Nursing
3525 Caroline Street
St. Louis, MO 63104

Components

The National Conference System is based on the PES format.

- □ P—the client's actual or potential problem
- □ E—the etiology or the factors contributing to the problem
- □ S—the signs and symptoms identified during the assessment phase

The nursing diagnosis is usually stated as a two part statement containing the problem and the etiology. The two parts of the diagnostic statement are joined by the words "related to," which implies a relationship between the problem and the etiology. The first part of the diagnosis, the problem *(P)*, is a clear, concise statement of the client's existing or potential health problem or unhealthful response. The problem is identified by the nurse during the assessment and diagnostic phases. This clause provides a clear indication of what needs to change. When identifying the unhealthful response, the nurse refers to the list of approved nursing diagnoses (Table 3–2).

The etiology *(E)* is the second part of the nursing diagnosis. The etiology is the environmental, sociocultural, psychological, physiological, or spiritual factors believed to be related to or contributing to the health problem. See Table 3–3 for examples of nursing diagnoses.

The *(S)* in the PES format stands for signs and symptoms identified during assessment. These are the cues that form the basis for nursing inferences and subsequent diagnoses. They are frequently documented in the data base or the nurses' notes.

Resource Books

Gordon (1982), Carpenito (1983), Kim et al (1984) and Duespohl (1986) have published books that are helpful in formulating nursing diagnoses according to the National Conference System. Each nursing diagnosis has a definition, etiological factors, and defining characteristics.

Issues Related to the National Conference System

Proponents of the National Conference System advocate its adoption as the universally accepted classification system. They argue that communication would be greatly enhanced if one system were used as the standard way of phrasing nursing diagnoses.

However, there are some difficulties associated with the National Conference System. The list of accepted nursing diagnoses is altered after each National Conference. Prior to 1982, the changes were based on

TABLE 3-2 □ APPROVED NURSING DIAGNOSES AT THE FIFTH NATIONAL CONFERENCE

Activity intolerance
Activity intolerance, potential
Airway clearance, ineffective
Anxiety
Bowel elimination, alteration in: constipation
Bowel elimination, alteration in: diarrhea
Bowel elimination, alteration in: incontinence
Breathing pattern, ineffective
Cardiac output, alteration in: decreased
Comfort, alteration in: pain
Communication, impaired: verbal
Coping, family: potential for growth
Coping, ineffective family: compromised
Coping, ineffective family: disabling
Coping, ineffective individual
Diversional activity, deficit
Family process, alteration in
Fear
Fluid volume, alteration in: excess
Fluid volume deficit, actual
Fluid volume deficit, potential
Gas exchange, impaired
Grieving, anticipatory
Grieving, dysfunctional
Health maintenance, alteration in
Home maintenance management, impaired
Injury: potential for
Knowledge deficit (specify)
Mobility, impaired physical
Noncompliance (specify)
Nutrition, alteration in: less than body requirements
Nutrition, alteration in: more than body requirements
Nutrition, alteration in: potential for more than body requirements
Oral mucous membrane, alteration in
Parenting, alteration in: actual or potential
Powerlessness
Rape trauma syndrome
Self-care deficit: feeding, bathing/hygiene, dressing/grooming, toileting
Self-concept, disturbance in: body image, self-esteem, role performance, personal
    identity
Sensory-perceptual alteration: visual, auditory, kinesthetic, gustatory, tactile, ol-
    factory
Sexual dysfunction
Skin integrity, impairment of: actual
Skin integrity, impairment of: potential
Sleep pattern disturbance
Social isolation
Spiritual distress (distress of the human spirit)
Thought processes, alteration in
Tissue perfusion, alteration in: cerebral, cardiopulmonary, renal, gastrointestinal,
    peripheral
Urinary elimination, alteration in patterns
Violence, potential for: self-directed or directed at others

From McLane A, McFarland K, and Kim M (eds): Classification of Nursing Diagnoses: Proceedings of the Fifth National Conference. St. Louis, CV Mosby, 1984, 470–471.

TABLE 3–3 □ **NATIONAL CONFERENCE SYSTEM—EXAMPLES OF NURSING DIAGNOSES**

Impaired verbal communication related to language barrier
Potential for injury related to impaired perception
Sexual dysfunction related to fear of rejection
Diversional activity deficit related to prolonged isolation
Ineffective individual coping related to lack of support systems
Knowledge deficit (insulin injection) related to lack of prior exposure to the procedure
Potential impairment of skin integrity related to irritating stomal drainage
Fear related to unknown etiology

opinion rather than on research. NANDA, recognizing that these frequent changes were frustrating to nurses in practice and education, made a new policy that future changes in approved nursing diagnoses are to be based on research.

Another concern with the National Conference System is that some of the nursing diagnoses are medically worded, describing problems that nurses would be hesitant to treat independently. Examples of these include "alteration in tissue perfusion," "fluid volume deficit," and "ineffective breathing pattern."

Marjory Gordon (1979) stated that the diagnosis "alteration in cardiac output" provides a good example of the need to define the nursing problem further. If the client has a disease that has altered cardiac output, what are the associated nursing problems? Are they anxiety, self-care deficit related to decreased activity tolerance, sleep pattern disturbance related to nocturnal dyspnea? There are many other possible nursing problems associated with alterations in cardiac output. In this case, it would be clearer to use a nursing diagnosis that would address the specific problems of the client.

The language used in the National Conference System has been described as vague, confusing, and inconsistent. It is expected that as the group continues to meet, it will recommend changes to clarify existing labels and suggest additions to the approved list.

Margaret Lunney (1982) has proposed a system to simplify the wording of the National Conference System. A complete description of her system appears in Appendix D.

An additional objection to the National Conference System is the absence of positive or strength-oriented nursing diagnoses. The vast majority of nursing diagnoses might be considered negative, since they focus on client's responses to illness rather than to health. Positive nursing diagnoses would communicate the client's strengths so that nurses could encourage their maintenance. The Fourth National Conference on Classification of Nursing Diagnoses accepted one positive nursing diagnosis—"Coping, family: potential for growth." This may pave the way for more positive nursing diagnoses in the future.

Public health nurses have asserted that, in addition to the absence of positive nursing diagnoses, the National Conference System does not adequately address their area of practice. The Omaha Classification Scheme, described in Appendix E, is an alternate system that fills the needs of many community health nurses.

Computer-Assisted Diagnosis

Computers are being used by physicians and nurses to organize and process data collected during assessment. Computer systems designed to assist in clinical diagnoses of disease and make recommendations about treatments are known as computer-assisted diagnosis (CAD) systems. "Although such systems are principally designed for use by physicians, nurses will have an increasing degree of interaction with them in the near future, as CAD systems become more readily available" (Andreoli and Musser, 1985).

The data collected from histories, examinations, and tests are entered into the computer. The computer may suggest possible diagnoses, additional tests to be ordered, and treatments found to be effective with the client's disease. Studies have shown that use of CAD leads to more thorough history-taking, improved accuracy and speed of diagnoses, better physician compliance with established treatment protocols, and more rational ordering of tests and diagnostic procedures (Tamarisk, 1982).

Computer-assisted nursing diagnosis involves the use of the computer to organize nursing assessment data. After the initial assessment data are entered, the computer draws up a list of actual, potential, and possible nursing diagnoses. The care plan created for each diagnosis may be altered to individualize it for the client. Figure 3–1 demonstrates a sample of a nursing diagnosis generated from a nursing assessment.

The chief advantages of computer-assisted nursing diagnosis center on the computer's ability to spot patterns that the nurse might overlook. The computer will not be affected by distraction, fatigue, headaches, or any of the other human variables that affect data processing.

The ability of the computer to generate nursing diagnoses is only as good as the program on which it is based. Lack of clinical knowledge on the part of the programmer can result in inaccurate diagnoses. Also, some nursing diagnoses simply lack large reliable data bases. Additionally, clients can display an infinite variety of responses to health problems,

```
DFALT-0981          NYUMC HOSP 4
05/28/85 11:55 AM                    PAGE 001

============================================
DEMONSTRATION DAN-1      1336
43~2877  85464  04/02/40   44 M
MARKS CLEMENT MD
============================================
```

```
                                          00000   000   00000
                                          0   0    0    0    0
                                          00000    0    00000
                                          0        0    0   0
                                          0       000    0
                                          ====================
                                          DEMONSTRATION DAN-1
```

```
PRIMARY DIAGNOSIS:  GI BLEED...

NURSING DIAGNOSIS
 05/22  ACTUAL SKIN BREAKDOWN R/T....INCONTINENCE OF URINE/FECES    JBKA
EXPECTED OUTCOMES                                      R/P    R/D
 05/22  DECREASE IN SIZE OF DECUBITUS ULCER            QD     5/30   JBKA
NURSING ORDERS
 05/22  TURN & POSITION Q2H                                          JBKA
 05/22  FOLLOW SCHEDULE--RT-BACK-LT                                  JBKA
 05/22  DO NOT ELEVATE HOB MORE THAN 30 DEG                          JBKA
 05/22  USE APPROPRIATE PRESSURE-RELIEVING DEVICE:
        WATER MATTRESS                                               JBKA
 05/22  OOB IN STRETCHER CHAIR TID                                   JBKA
 05/22  PAD BEDPAN                                                   JBKA
 05/22  PASSIVE ROM TO ALL EXTREMITIES Q4H                          JBKA
 05/22  DIETARY CONSULT REGARDING ASSESSMENT OF
        NUTRITIONAL STATUS                                          JBKA
 05/22  CHECK FOR FECAL/URINARY INCONTINENCE
        Q1/2H. (NA TO CHECK Q1H ON THE 1/2H & RN TO
        CHECK Q1H ON THE HOUR)                                      JBKA
 05/22  CLEAN SKIN THOROUGHLY & PAT DRY POST VOID/BM                 JBKA
 05/22  METHOD OF TREATMENT: STAGE 3- STOMA ADHESIVE
        METHOD                                                      JBKA
 05/22  WEAR STERILE GLOVES WHEN IN CONTACT W/
        WOUND.
        CLEANSE AREA, USING A STERILE IRRIG TRAY W/
        1/2 STRENGTH PEROXIDE & NS.
        RINSE THOROUGHLY W/ NS & PAT DRY W/ STERILE
        GAUZE                                                       JBKA
 05/22  APPLY HEAT LAMP X15 MINS 12 INCHES FROM SKIN
        & AT THE SIDE OF BED SO THAT INADVERTENT PT
        MOVEMENT WILL NOT CAUSE LAMP TO CONTACT
        SKIN.
        PAT ANTACID OVER THE AFFECTED AREA USING
        STERILE GAUZE. ALLOW TO DRY THOROUGHLY                      JBKA
 05/22  APPLY MYCOSTATIN POWDER AS ORDERED BY MD.
        REMOVE EXCESS POWDER BY BRUSHING W/ STERILE
        GAUZE.
        APPLY A LIGHT COAT OF SKIN PREP. ALLOW AREA
        TO DRY THOROUGHLY                                           JBKA
 05/22  APPLY STOMA ADHESIVE TO COVER THE ENTIRE
        AREA EXTENDING 1 INCH BEYOND THE REDNESS ON
        ALL SIDES. ROUND THE CORNERS W/ A SCISSOR TO
        PREVENT WRINKLING.
        SECURE THE EDGES OF THE STOMA ADHESIVE W/ 1
        INCH PAPER TAPE                                             JBKA
 05/22  LEAVE DSG IN PLACE 2-3 DAYS IF THE INTEGRITY

                          CONTINUED
============================================================
DEMONSTRATION DAN-1                     PATIENT CARE PLAN
```

Figure 3–1 □ Computer sample of nursing diagnosis. (Courtesy of New York University Medical Center)

Illustration continued on following page

```
05/28/85  11:55 AM              PAGE  002
                                                  00000   000   00000
                                                  0   0   0   0   0   0
========================================          00000   0     00000
DEMONSTRATION DAN-1        1336                    0       0   0   0
4342877  85464   04/02/40   44  M                  0       000    0
MARKS CLEMENT MD                                  ================  ===
========================================          DEMONSTRATION DAN-1
```

        OF THE DSG REMAINS INTACT   EKA

                          LAST PAGE

Figure 3–1 *Continued*

making it difficult to anticipate all such responses. Nurses using computers for diagnosis need to exercise professional judgment in evaluating the conclusions reached by the computer.

SUMMARY

After data are collected during the assessment phase, they are organized, interpreted, and validated. These steps can be affected by several types of errors, including inaccurate or incomplete data, inaccurate interpretation of data, and lack of clinical knowledge or experience. Errors can result in nursing diagnoses that are not accurate.

Nursing diagnoses are used to communicate the client's problems and related etiologies. While there are several objections to nursing diagnoses, many benefits are associated with their use. These include providing a focus for the nursing process, identifying the scope of nursing practice, and communicating in nursing's professional language. The National Conference System is used most commonly to achieve these purposes. It provides a format for the era of computer-assisted nursing diagnoses.

References

American Nurses' Association: Standards of Practice. Kansas City, MO: American Nurses' Association, 1973.

American Nurses' Association: Nursing: A Social Policy Statement. Kansas City, MO: American Nurses' Association, 1980.

Andreoli K and Musser L: Computers in nursing care: the state of the art. Nursing Outlook 33(1): 16–25, 1985.

Carpenito L: Nursing Diagnosis: Application to Clinical Practice. Philadelphia: JB Lippincott, 1983.

Confidentially. Nursing '83, 70, January 1983a.

Confidentially. Nursing '83, 94, April 1983b.

Confidentially. Nursing '84, 72, December 1984.

Confidentially. Nursing '85, 33, February 1985.

Cushing M: First, anticipate the harm . . . American Journal of Nursing 137–138, February 1985.

Duesphol A: Nursing Diagnosis Handbook. Philadelphia: WB Saunders, 1986.

Gaines B and McFarland M: Nursing diagnosis: its relationship and use in nursing education. In Nursing Diagnosis, Topics in Clinical Nursing, 39–49, January 1984.

Gordon, M: Nursing diagnoses and the diagnostic process. American Journal of Nursing 76(8):1298–1300, 1976.

Gordon M: The concept of nursing diagnosis. Nursing Clinics of North America, 14(3):487–495, September 1979.

Gordon, M: Manual of Nursing Diagnoses. New York: McGraw-Hill, 1982.

Kim M, McFarland G, McLane A: Pocket Guide to Nursing Diagnosis. St. Louis: CV Mosby, 1984.

Lunney M: Nursing diagnosis: refining the system. American Journal of Nursing 456–459, March 1982.

Moritz D: Nursing diagnoses in relation to the nursing process. In Moritz D and Kim M (eds): Classification of Nursing Diagnoses: Proceedings of the Third and Fourth National Conferences. New York: McGraw-Hill, 1982, 53–57.

Mundinger M and Jauron G: Developing a nursing diagnosis. Nursing Outlook 33(2)94–98, 1975.
Tamarisk N: The computer as a clinical tool. Nursing Management 46–49, August 1982.

Bibliography

Abdellah F, Martin A, Beland I, and Matheney R: Patient Centered Approaches to Nursing. New York: Macmillan, 1960.
Andrews P: Nursing diagnoses. In Griffith J and Christensen P: Nursing Process. St. Louis: CV Mosby, 1982.
Aspinall M: Nursing diagnosis—the weak link. Nursing Outlook 24(7):433–437, July 1976.
Baer C: Nursing diagnoses: a futuristic process for nursing practice. In Nursing Diagnosis, Topics in Clinical Nursing, 89–96, January 1984.
Block D: Some crucial terms in nursing—what do they really mean? Nursing Outlook, 22(11):689–694, November 1974.
Bockrath M: Your patient needs two diagnoses—medical and nursing. Nursing Life, 29–32, March/April 1982.
Brooks E: The starting point. Nursing Management 35–37, June 1983.
Bruce J: Implementation of nursing diagnoses. Nursing Clinics of North America 14(3):509–515, September 1979.
Bumbalo J and Sieman M: Nursing assessment and diagnosis: mental health problems of children. Topics in Clinical Nursing 41–54, April 1983.
Davidson S: Nursing diagnosis: its application in the acute care setting. Nursing Diagnosis, Topics in Clinical Nursing, 50–56, January 1984.
delBueno D, Demers B, Isler C, et al: What's your diagnosis? RN 104:63–71, 1980.
Dossey B and Guzzetta C: Nursing diagnoses. Nursing '81, 34–38, June 1981.
Feild L: The implementation of nursing diagnoses in clinical practice. Nursing Clinics of North America 14(3):497–508, 1979.
Fortin J and Rabinow J: Legal implications of nursing diagnoses. Nursing Clinics of North America 14:(3):553–561, 1979.
Fredette S and Gloriant F: Nursing diagnoses in cancer chemotherapy. American Journal of Nursing 2013–2022, November 1981.
Fry V: The creative approach to nursing. American Journal of Nursing 53(3):301–302, 1953.
Fuhs M: It seems like acute respiratory dysfunction. RN 51–54, October 1979.
Gerber F: Diabetes out of control. RN 65–68, September 1979.
Gordon M: Nursing Diagnoses—Process and Application. New York: McGraw-Hill, 1982.
Gordon M: Report of the task force conference group of classification of nursing diagnoses. In McLane A, McFarland K, and Kim M (eds): Classification of Nursing Diagnoses: Proceedings of the Fifth National Conference. St. Louis: CV Mosby, 1984, 548–552.
Gordon M, McKeehan K, and Sweeney M: Nursing diagnosis: look at its use in the clinical area. American Journal of Nursing 672–674, April 1980.
Kim M and McFarland G: Analysis of view on issues and trends related to nursing diagnoses and the national conference. In McLane A, McFarland K, and Kim M (eds): Classification of Nursing Diagnoses: Proceedings of the Fifth National Conference. St. Louis: CV Mosby, 1984, 556–570.
Lucas C and Young M: Nursing diagnosis: common problems in implementation. Nursing Diagnosis, Topics of Clinical Nursing 68–77, January 1984.
Popkess S: Diagnosing your patient's strengths. Nursing '81 34–37, July 1981.
Popkess-Vawter S: Strength oriented nursing diagnoses. In McLane A, McFarland K, and Kim M (eds): Classification of Nursing Diagnoses: Proceedings of the Fifth National Conference. St. Louis: CV Mosby, 1984, 433–440.
Roy SC: A diagnostic classification system for nursing. Nursing Outlook 23(2):90–94, 1975.
Shoemaker J: How nursing diagnosis helps focus your care. RN 56–61, August 1979.
Tilton C and Maloof M: Diagnosing the problems in stroke. American Journal of Nursing 596–601, April 1982.

4

How to Write A Nursing Diagnosis

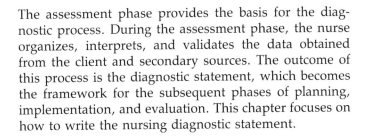

The assessment phase provides the basis for the diagnostic process. During the assessment phase, the nurse organizes, interprets, and validates the data obtained from the client and secondary sources. The outcome of this process is the diagnostic statement, which becomes the framework for the subsequent phases of planning, implementation, and evaluation. This chapter focuses on how to write the nursing diagnostic statement.

COMPONENTS OF THE DIAGNOSTIC STATEMENT

A nursing diagnostic statement consists of two parts joined by the phrase "related to." In writing nursing diagnoses, the nurse should remember that the diagnostic statement *begins with a determination of the **problem** of the client* (Part I) and *identifies the **etiology** (contributing factors)* (Part II).

Part I—The Problem

The first part of the statement specifies the problem identified by the nurse during the assessment phase.

This clause provides a clear indication of what needs to change and determines the goals that will measure the change.

When writing the first part, the nurse should consider two areas.

1. What is the problem that is inferred by assessment data?
2. To what degree is the problem present?

The problem can be determined by considering the list of accepted nursing diagnoses (see Table 3–2).

Modifiers

Qualifying phrases precede or follow the problem to identify stages or levels. As can be seen in Table 3–2, colons or comas separate the various parts of the first clause of the diagnosis.

Examples of Modifiers

☐ Alteration in—a change from the usual optimum for a particular client. For example, a client who is hallucinating has a diagnosis of "alteration in thought processes."
☐ Potential—the individual is at risk for a problem. For example, a blind client may have a diagnosis of "potential for injury."
☐ Possible—the problem may be present, but more data need to be collected and validated. For example, a nurse observes a mother visiting her hospitalized two year old. The mother acts cool and distant toward the child. The nurse writes a diagnosis of "possible alteration in parenting" and plans to gather more data to validate the diagnosis.

Additional Modifiers		Examples
Acute	Chronic	Acute anxiety
Excess	Deficit	Fluid volume deficit
Increased	Decreased	Alteration in cardiac output: decreased
Less than	More than	Alteration in nutrition, more than body requirements
Dysfunctional		Dysfunctional grieving
Impaired		Impaired physical mobility
Ineffective		Ineffective airway clearance
Compromised		Ineffective family coping: compromised
Disabling		Ineffective family coping: disabling
Disturbance in		Disturbance in self-concept

Example. Mrs. James is a 72 year old client who had a total hip replacement this morning for chronic arthritis. During your assessment, she complains of postoperative incisional pain and mentions her concern about becoming constipated.

This information suggests two nursing diagnoses that reflect comfort and elimination concerns. The first parts would be written

1. Alteration in comfort: pain   indicates that the client is experiencing discomfort

2. Potential alteration in bowel elimination: constipation   reflects the client's concern about the possibility that she will become constipated

Part II—The Etiology

The etiology constitutes the second clause of the nursing diagnosis. To prevent, minimize, or alleviate the problem, the nurse must know why it is occurring. The etiology reflects the environmental, psychological, sociocultural, physiological, or spiritual factors believed to be related or contributing to the health problem.

Examples of Etiological Factors

Environmental	Psychological
Excessive noise	Fear of death
Noxious odors	Feelings of loneliness
Sensitivity to light	Impaired parental-infant bonding

Sociocultural	Physiological
Inability to procure food	Swallowing difficulties
Language barrier	Sensory deficit
Lack of support systems	Abnormal fluid loss

Spiritual
Inability to practice religious rituals
Challenged beliefs about God
Conflict between religious beliefs and prescribed health regimen

In the preceding case of Mrs. James, two problems were suggested. The second parts could be written as follows.

Problem	Etiology
1. Alteration in comfort: pain	effects of surgery
2. Potential alteration in bowel elimination: constipation	prolonged immobility

Remember that the etiology helps to identify specific nursing interventions that will prevent, correct, or alleviate the problem. For example, the following diagnoses have the same problem but quite different etiologies.

Problem	related to	Etiology
1. Alteration in nutrition (less than body requirements)		difficulty in swallowing
2. Alteration in nutrition (less than body requirements)		anorexia
3. Alteration in nutrition (less than body requirements)		feelings of loneliness

The nursing interventions suggested by each of these diagnoses are also quite different. Those to be used in the presence of swallowing difficulties might be as follows.
1. Sit the client in an upright position, 60 to 90°
2. Encourage the client to

☐ take small amounts of semisolid foods
☐ place food at the back of the mouth
☐ think about swallowing

If the client is experiencing anorexia, the following interventions may help.
1. Determine food likes and dislikes
2. Serve food in an appealing manner
3. Provide small, frequent feedings

For the client who does not eat because she is lonely following her husband's death, the nurse may include these interventions.
1. Encourage the client to verbalize feelings about the death of her husband
2. Explain the hazards of continued decreased intake
3. Arrange consultation with a psychiatric clinical specialist
4. Provide information about support groups—Widows & Widowers, I Can Cope.

Summary of the Components of the Diagnostic Statement

Figure 4–1 illustrates the relationship of the components of a nursing diagnostic statement.

Note that qualifying statements may be added to increase the clarity of a diagnosis (e.g., constipation vs. diarrhea). Also, closely related etiological factors may be grouped within the diagnostic statement (e.g., immobility and side effects of codeine). The nursing orders include interventions or specific approaches to deal with each factor.

VARIATIONS OF THE DIAGNOSTIC STATEMENT

A problem may be related to more than one etiological factor. For example, "potential alteration in bowel elimination: constipation" can be related to prolonged immobility, decreased oral intake, and change in diet.

At times, the second part of the nursing diagnosis, or the etiology, is itself broken into two parts, using the words "secondary to" or the abbreviation "2°."

Examples

Fluid volume deficit related to decreased consumption of oral fluids secondary to weakness
Alteration in nutrition less than body requirements related to decreased appetite 2° loss of child

As can be seen above, the two parts of the diagnostic statement are usually joined by the words "related to." A few nursing diagnoses will be written as a one-part statement without the words "related to" or an identified etiology. An example is "rape trauma syndrome," in which the etiology is obvious. In general, it is not desirable to leave out the etiology because it directs the interventions.

At times, the etiology will be unclear or unknown. It is acceptable to describe the problem using the words "related to unknown etiology" while continuing to search for the etiology.

Example. Alteration in comfort: pain related to unknown etiology.

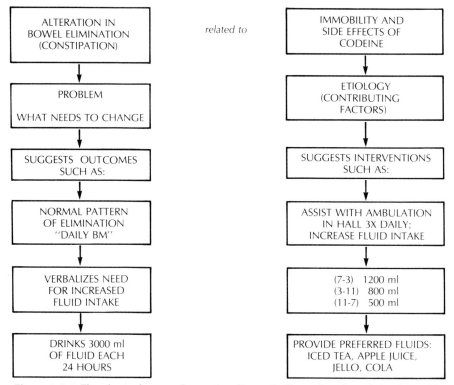

Figure 4–1 □ Flowchart of a sample nursing diagnosis illustrating the relationship of its components.

MEDICAL VERSUS NURSING DIAGNOSES

The nursing diagnostic statement differs from the medical diagnosis, since it reflects the essence of nursing rather than medical practice. The following outline sets forth the primary differences between medical and nursing diagnoses.

Medical	Nursing
Identifies a specific illness	Identifies an actual or potential response to the illness
Clinical manifestations suggest a medical need	Responses suggest a nursing need
Implies associated medical interventions	Implies associated nursing interventions

The examples below are a comparison of medical and nursing diagnoses.

Medical Diagnosis	Nursing Diagnosis
Hepatitis	Ineffective individual coping related to prolonged isolation
Diabetes mellitus	Knowledge deficit (foot care) related to inability to recall information received in the past
Cancer	Alteration in oral mucous membranes related to effects of chemotherapy
Myocardial infarction	Disturbance in self-concept: self-esteem related to change in role
Hemorrhagic stroke	Potential for injury related to motor deficit (right-sided weakness)

GUIDELINES FOR WRITING A NURSING DIAGNOSIS

Formulation of a nursing diagnostic statement may be considered a new skill. Just like any other new skill, it takes practice. The nurse will find that, with practice, the process of writing nursing diagnoses becomes easier.

One way to reduce frustration is to utilize the following guidelines when developing the diagnostic statement.

1. Write the Diagnosis in Terms of Response Rather Than Need

The first part of the diagnostic statement identifies the client's response to illness or state of health. Therapeutic or functional needs, such as "needs frequent turning" or "needs coughing and deep breathing," describe nursing interventions rather than health responses and therefore should not be included in the first part of the diagnostic statement.

Example. Mrs. Jane Suydam has a nasogastric tube and cannot have anything by mouth. She expresses the fact that her mouth and lips are dry. The nurse decides that the client "needs mouth care." The nurse concludes that she is uncomfortable because of dry mucous membranes caused by lack of fluid intake and mouth breathing. The nurse communicates Jane's problem via the nursing care plan in the diagnostic statement "alteration in comfort related to dry oral mucous membranes."

Examples

Incorrect	Correct
Needs adequate nutrition	Potential alteration in nutrition greater than body requirements related to excessive caloric intake
Needs frequent turning	Impaired mobility related to left-sided weakness

2. Use "Related to" Rather than "Due to" or "Caused by"

The two parts of the diagnostic statement should always be linked together by the words "related to." This identifies a relationship between the problem and the etiology and implies that if one part of the diagnosis changes, the other part may also change. "Related to" does not necessarily mean that there is direct cause and effect between the two parts. When such phrases as "due to" or "caused by" are used, the second part of the diagnostic statement could be interpreted as the specific cause of the problem.

Example

Potential for injury caused by change in mental status	Potential for injury related to change in mental status

In reality, the nurse may be unaware of other contributing factors that are influencing the problem.

Example. Mrs. Arlene Dillione is three days post-op after a mastectomy for cancer of the breast. The nurse has identified the change in body image as a contributing factor in her alteration in coping. Writing this diagnostic statement as "ineffective coping due to change in body image" implies that the mastectomy is the cause of Arlene's alteration in coping. In validating this diagnosis, the nurse discovers that Arlene's mother died one month before from cancer of the breast. A more appropriate nursing diagnostic statement is "ineffective coping related to change in body image and grieving process."

3. Write the Diagnosis in Legally Advisable Terms

A diagnostic statement such as "potential impairment of skin integrity related to infrequent turning" is not legally advisable. This statement implies negligence or blame, which can create potential legal problems for the personnel caring for the client. This statement could be better phrased as "potential impairment of skin integrity related to decreased mobility." The therapeutic nursing orders would be similar in both instances, but the second statement is factual and does not imply fault.

Examples

Incorrect	Correct
Potential for injury related to inadequately maintained skin traction	Potential for injury related to hazards of skin traction
Ineffective airway clearance related to inadequate suction	Ineffective airway clearance related to effects of sedation

4. Write the Diagnosis without Value Judgments

Nursing diagnoses should be based on objective and subjective data collected and validated in cooperation with the client or significant other. The behavior of the client should not be judged by the nurse's personal values and standards. The use of words such as inadequate, poor, and unhealthy frequently imply value judgments.

Examples

Incorrect	Correct
Alteration in parenting related to poor bonding with child	Alteration in parenting related to prolonged separation from child
Impaired home maintenance management related to poor housekeeping habits, cluttered household	Impaired home maintenance management related to lack of knowledge regarding home safety measures

5. Avoid Reversing the Clauses

Remember that the first part of the diagnostic statement reflects the problem and defines outcomes. The second part of the statement defines the etiology and suggests nursing orders. Reversing the clauses may result in unclear communication about the client's problem and its etiology. This would make it difficult to write appropriate outcomes and nursing orders.

Examples

Incorrect	Correct
Disorientation related to sleep pattern disturbance	Sleep pattern disturbance related to disorientation
Decreased caloric intake related to alteration in nutrition (less than body requirements)	Alteration in nutrition (less than body requirements) related to decreased caloric intake

6. Avoid Including Signs and Symptoms of Illness in the First Part of the Statement

The first part of the diagnostic statement is derived from a cluster of signs and symptoms observed by the nurse during the assessment of the client. An isolated sign or symptom is not a nursing diagnosis, but it may provide cues to help identify the problem. Inaccurate diagnoses may occur if the nurse focuses on an isolated sign or symptom rather than the entire clinical picture.

Example. William Ward, an elderly client admitted to a nursing home, has a history of emphysema. The nurse observes that he is restless. Writing the diagnosis as "restlessness related to change in level of consciousness" suggests that restlessness is the problem. In fact, the presence of restlessness may be a cue to other responses, such as ineffective airway clearance, alterations in coping, or fear.

7. The First Part of the Diagnosis Should Only Include Problems

In some instances, clients express feelings regarding their illness or environment that are not necessarily unexpected or problematic. For instance, anger may be an expected client response at a certain point in the process of recovery.

Example. Tony Smith is an 18 year old college freshman on a sports scholarship at Princeton University. During semester break in Bermuda, he was involved in a motor bike accident, resulting in the traumatic amputation of his right leg. In the course of his hospitalization, Tony expresses his anger verbally and physically. He slams his fist down on the mattress and screams at the nurses. His anger is not necessarily inappropriate at this point in his recovery. Therefore it would not be valid to write a nursing diagnosis of "ineffective coping related to feelings of anger." Later, Tony refuses physical therapy and dressing changes and tries to strike the nurses. At this point, his anger does represent ineffective coping, since it interferes with his recovery and rehabilitation.

8. Be Sure that the Two Parts of the Diagnosis Do Not Mean the Same Thing

In some instances, diagnostic statements are written in which the two clauses say the same thing. Examine this statement: "alteration in breath sounds related to rhonchi in left lung." Both parts of the statement have the same meaning. In reality, the client is experiencing a problem in airway clearance. The diagnostic statement should be written as "ineffective airway clearance related to retained secretions."

Examples

Incorrect	Correct
Inability to feed self related to feeding problems	Self-care deficit: feeding, related to pain in fingers
Impairment of skin integrity related to broken area of skin	Impairment of skin integrity related to prolonged immobility

9. The Problem or Etiological Factors Should Be Expressed in Terms that Can Be Changed

Keep in mind that the diagnostic statement identifies actual or potential problems. These problems and the factors that contribute to their presence should be changeable by intervention within the realm of nursing practice.

Example. Shelby Donovan is a six year old who is two days post-op after an appendectomy. She is crying and points to the incisional area and says, "My tummy hurts." The diagnosis "alteration in comfort: pain related to surgical incision" is not accurate because nursing intervention cannot change the presence of a surgical incision. This can be restated as "alteration in comfort: pain related to effects of surgery." Nursing interventions may relieve the effects of surgery—pain, immobility, anxiety, nausea.

Examples

Incorrect	Correct
Knowledge deficit related to pregnancy	Knowledge deficit related to prenatal diet
Alteration in urinary elimination related to enlarged prostate gland	Alteration in urinary elmination related to incontinence

10. The Medical Diagnosis Should Not Be Included in the Nursing Diagnostic Statement

Two types of errors are commonly seen involving the medical diagnosis. The first is the use of the medical diagnosis in either of the two parts of the nursing diagnosis. Since the medical diagnosis suggests medical interventions, its use is inappropriate in a nursing diagnosis.

Examples

Incorrect	Correct
Ineffective breathing pattern related to emphysema	Ineffective breathing pattern related to retained secretions
Diabetes related to obesity	Alteration in health maintenance related to excessive caloric intake

The second type of error is a tendency to write the nursing diagnosis as a paraphrased medical diagnosis. For example, a patient with hypertension may be given a nursing diagnosis of "alteration in circulation related to pressure changes." This is simply a restatement of the medical diagnosis. The purpose of nursing diagnoses is to keep the focus on the whole client and to examine the client's problems that are within the domain of nursing.

Case Study

Jose Esposito is a 56 year old office worker who is admitted with a diagnosis of hypertension and a blood pressure of 170/110 mm Hg. When questioned about medications, he admits that he had a prescription for an antihypertensive medication, but he stopped taking it when he finished the bottle two weeks ago. "It interfered with my sex life, and I thought I could do without the medication," he said. From this small amount of data, it is possible to derive two nursing diagnoses that are more explicit than the medical diagnosis of hypertension: (1) knowledge deficit related to importance of medication, and (2) sexual dysfunction related to side effects of antihypertensive medication.

Although there is overlap in the nursing and medical professions, the purpose of nursing diagnosis is to keep the planning of care focused on problems that are amenable to nursing interventions.

PITFALLS IN WRITING NURSING DIAGNOSES

Student and graduate nurses who are learning how to write nursing diagnoses are sometimes puzzled about how to handle certain common situations. These situations include the identification of more than one problem or etiological factor and how to avoid writing wordy nursing diagnoses.

More Than One Problem

At times the nurse identifies several actual or potential problems that are related to the same etiology.

Example. Gita Raman delivers a premature baby who is placed in the high-risk nursery for intensive care. As a result of being separated from her infant, Gita experiences anxiety. She says to the nursery nurse, "I'm afraid to touch the baby. I might hurt her."

A nursing diagnosis for Gita could be "ineffective coping and parenting related to disruption in maternal-infant bonding." One potential pitfall in writing a nursing diagnosis with two problems as the first part is the possibility of overlooking appropriate outcomes for each problem. The outcomes for each of these problems are quite different.

Ineffective Coping	Alteration in Parenting
As a result of nursing interventions, within 48 hours Gita will:	As a result of nursing interventions, within 24 hours Gita will:
□ Verbalize positive feelings about maternal abilities □ Begin to establish rapport with parents of other premature infants	□ Touch her baby □ Call her by name □ Make positive comments about her baby □ Maintain eye contact with her baby

The nursing diagnosis for Gita could be revised by separating it into two diagnoses: "ineffective coping related to feelings of anxiety" and "alteration in parenting related to disruption of maternal-infant bonding." This separation encourages development of specific goals for each problem. In addition, the time-frame for resolution may be different for each response. Therefore, separation of the diagnoses facilitates individual outcomes evaluation.

Example. While the nurse is changing the dressing on Murray Heston's amputation stump, the 48 year old man looks sadly at his leg. "Did you know that in my younger days I was in the Boston Marathon? But look at me! I'm a good for nothing cripple. I can't even get myself into a wheelchair. Makes me wonder what my wife really thinks of me now."

The nursing diagnosis for Murray could be "disturbance in self-concept: self-esteem, and ineffective coping related to fear of rejection, change in body image, and feelings of helplessness." This could be broken down into two separate nursing diagnoses with outcomes for each.

Disturbance in self-concept: self-esteem, related to change in body image and feelings of helplessness	Ineffective coping related to fear of rejection

Outcomes	Outcomes
By time of discharge:	By time of discharge:

By time of discharge:

☐ Continues to verbalize his concerns about change in body image
☐ Independently transfers himself from bed to wheelchair
☐ Identifies resources to use for rehabilitation process

By time of discharge:

☐ Reports that he has discussed his concerns with wife
☐ Identifies support system

More Than One Etiological Factor

Another question that frequently arises is what to do if more than one factor relates to the first part of the nursing diagnosis. Clients' health care problems are rarely simple. There are frequently several factors that contribute to an illness. This is illustrated in the case of Jose Esposito, who has hypertension and discontinued his medication because it interfered with his sex life. When Jose is admitted to the hospital, his weight is recorded as 170 lb. He is 5 ft, 4 in. In reviewing what Jose eats in a normal day, the nurse determines that his caloric intake is excessive. His favorite leisure activities are watching TV and drinking beer. "I know I need to lose weight, but I've never had any success in the past, so I've given up trying." He smokes two to three packs of cigarettes a day.

With these data, it is possible to expand on the nursing diagnosis of "alteration in health maintenance" to include some additional factors: "alteration in health maintenance related to lack of knowledge of the effects of medication, smoking, and obesity on hypertension."

Another nursing diagnosis for Jose could be stated as: "alteration in nutrition: more than body requirements related to excessive caloric intake and sedentary lifestyle."

In Jose's case, his obesity, sedentary lifestyle, smoking, and discontinuation of the antihypertensive medication are all contributing to his hypertension, which illustrates the complex nature of his illness. Linkage of two or more factors with the first part of the nursing diagnosis creates a more compact nursing diagnosis. Imagine how redundant it would be if Jose's nursing diagnoses were written as

"Alteration in health maintenance related to lack of knowledge of effects of medication on hypertension."

"Alteration in health maintenance related to lack of knowledge of effects of smoking and obesity on hypertension."

"Alteration in nutrition: more than body requirements related to excessive caloric intake."

"Alteration in nutrition: more than body requirements related to sedentary lifestyle."

Clearly it is more concise to group closely related factors within one nursing diagnosis. For example

"Alteration in health maintenance related to lack of knowledge of effects of medication, smoking, and obesity on hypertension."

"Alteration in nutrition: more than body requirements related to excessive caloric intake and sedentary lifestyle."

Wordy Nursing Diagnoses

The nursing diagnoses should be stated clearly and concisely, since wordy statements tend to obscure the focus.

Example. Gita Raman, the mother of a premature baby, reveals that she feels that she caused her premature labor. "I wouldn't be in this mess if I hadn't lifted a can of paint—that's why my labor started."

A nursing diagnosis for Gita might be phrased as "ineffective coping related to belief that she caused the onset of premature labor by lifting paint can on the day of delivery."

Although the client's comments are cues that suggest her feelings of guilt, it is not necessary to include her statement verbatim in the nursing diagnosis. This diagnosis could be expressed clearly and concisely as "ineffective coping related to feelings of guilt."

Gita also reveals that she is concerned about her two year old son, since she spends the majority of her day at the hospital. She also sees very little of her husband, and this has created tension in their marriage. The nursing diagnosis could be worded "alteration in the interactions between husband and wife and mother and two year old son related to mother's hospital visiting patterns." However, the diagnosis could be more concisely stated as "alteration in family process related to mother's hospital visiting pattern."

Clear, concise diagnostic statements facilitate communication and allow the nurse to concentrate on those factors contributing to the existence of a specific problem. This approach promotes quality individualized nursing care.

VERIFICATION OF THE DIAGNOSIS

Before committing the diagnosis to paper, it is helpful to verify its accuracy. This can be accomplished by the nurse's asking the following questions.

☐ Is the data base sufficient and accurate?
☐ Does a pattern exist?
☐ Are the signs and symptoms used to determine the existence of a pattern characteristic of the pattern identified?
☐ Is the nursing diagnosis based on nursing knowledge?
☐ Can the nursing diagnosis be altered by independent nursing actions?
☐ Would other nurses formulate the same nursing diagnosis based on the data? (Price, 1980.)

After asking all these questions, the nurse should, if possible, verify the diagnosis with the client by describing what the nurse perceives as the problems and asking if the client agrees. If agreement is not achieved, the nurse and the client continue to discuss the problem until consensus is reached.

DOCUMENTATION

After developing and verifying the nursing diagnosis, the nurse documents it on the chart and care plan. Specifically, it should be included on nurses' notes or progress notes, discharge summaries, and interagency referral forms. Diagnostic statements are reviewed at intervals and revised as necessary.

SUMMARY

To summarize, the assessment phase includes data collection, validation, and documentation. The diagnostic phase involves data processing and formulation of the nursing diagnosis. This chapter has presented guidelines for writing the diagnostic statement. The diagnosis is verified with the client and documented.

In review, here are the guidelines for writing nursing diagnoses.

1. Write the diagnosis in terms of response rather than need.
2. Use "related to" rather than "due to" or "caused by."
3. Write the diagnosis in legally advisable terms.
4. Write the diagnosis without value judgments.
5. Avoid reversing the clauses.
6. Avoid including signs and symptoms in the first part of the statement.
7. The first part of the diagnosis should only include problems.
8. Be sure that the two parts of the diagnosis do not mean the same thing.
9. The problem or etiological factors should be expressed in terms that can be changed.
10. The medical diagnosis should not be included in the nursing diagnostic statement.

4–1 TEST YOURSELF

IDENTIFICATION OF CORRECTLY AND INCORRECTLY WRITTEN DIAGNOSES

The following is a list of nursing diagnostic statements. Decide whether each statement is correctly or incorrectly written. If incorrectly stated, identify the rule(s) violated, by number, from the preceding list.

	Correct	Incorrect	Rule
1. Potential for injury due to cataract surgery and corneal transplant			
2. Alteration in comfort: pain related to arthritis			
3. Poor hygiene related to laziness			
4. Alteration in fluid volume: excess related to excessive sodium intake			
5. Inability to learn related to learning disability			
6. Needs skin care			
7. Spiritual distress related to separation from cultural ties			
8. Anger related to diagnosis of cancer			
9. Alteration in level of consciousness due to transient ischemic attack			
10. Alteration in nutrition (less than body requirements) related to lack of knowledge regarding diabetic exchange diet			
11. Dysfunctional grieving related to death of spouse			
12. Alteration in bodily functions related to vaginal secretions			
13. Activity intolerance related to chronic pain			
14. Social isolation related to unacceptable social behavior			
15. Sensory overload related to alteration in thought processes			
16. Ineffective breathing patterns related to pneumonia			
17. Alteration in temperature caused by infection			
18. Alteration in urinary elimination related to catheter obstruction			
19. Alteration in thought processes related to impaired thinking			
20. Potential for injury related to failure of nurses to put up side rails			

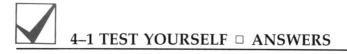

4–1 TEST YOURSELF □ ANSWERS

Guidelines for Writing Nursing Diagnoses
1. Write the diagnosis in terms of response rather than need.
2. Use "related to" rather than "due to" or "caused by."
3. Write the diagnosis in legally advisable terms.
4. Write the diagnosis without value judgments.
5. Avoid reversing the clauses.
6. Avoid including signs and symptoms in the first part of the statement.
7. The first part of the diagnosis should only include problems.
8. Be sure that the two parts of the diagnosis do not mean the same thing.
9. The problem or etiological factors should be expressed in terms that can be changed.
10. The medical diagnosis should not be included in the nursing diagnostic statement.

	Correct	Incorrect	Rule
1. Potential for injury due to cataract surgery and corneal transplant		✔	2, 9, 10
2. Alteration in comfort: pain related to arthritis		✔	10
3. Poor hygiene related to laziness		✔	4
4. Alteration in fluid volume: excess related to excessive sodium intake	✔		
5. Inability to learn related to learning disability		✔	8
6. Needs skin care		✔	1
7. Spiritual distress related to separation from cultural ties	✔		
8. Anger related to diagnosis of cancer		✔	7, 9
9. Alteration in level of consciousness due to transient ischemic attack		✔	2, 10
10. Alteration in nutrition (less than body requirements) related to lack of knowledge regarding diabetic exchange diet	✔		
11. Dysfunctional grieving related to death of spouse		✔	9
12. Alteration in bodily functions related to vaginal secretions		✔	6
13. Activity intolerance related to chronic pain	✔		
14. Social isolation related to unacceptable social behavior	✔		
15. Sensory overload related to alteration in thought processes		✔	5
16. Ineffective breathing patterns related to pneumonia		✔	10
17. Alteration in temperature caused by infection		✔	2, 6
18. Alteration in urinary elimination related to catheter obstruction	✔		
19. Alteration in thought processes related to impaired thinking		✔	8
20. Potential for injury related to failure of nurses to put up side rails		✔	3

✓ 4–2 TEST YOURSELF

REVISION OF INCORRECTLY WRITTEN DIAGNOSES

The nursing diagnoses that were incorrectly written are listed below. Revise each statement to make it correct.

Statement	Revised
1. Potential for injury due to cataract surgery and corneal transplant	
2. Alteration in comfort: pain related to arthritis	
3. Poor hygiene related to laziness	
4. Inability to learn related to learning disability	
5. Needs skin care	
6. Anger related to diagnosis of cancer	
7. Alteration in level of consciousness due to transient ischemic attack	
8. Dysfunctional grieving related to death of spouse	
9. Alteration in bodily functions related to vaginal secretions	
10. Sensory overload related to alteration in thought processes	
11. Ineffective breathing patterns related to pneumonia	
12. Alteration in temperature caused by infection	
13. Alteration in thought processes related to impaired thinking	
14. Potential for injury related to failure of nurses to put up side rails	
15. Alteration in nutrition (more than body requirements) related to poor eating habits	
16. Insomnia related to sleep pattern disturbance	

4–2 TEST YOURSELF □ ANSWERS

Statement	Revised	Comments
1. Potential for injury due to cataract surgery and corneal transplant	Potential for injury related to impaired perception (eye patch)	
2. Alteration in comfort: pain related to arthritis	Alteration in comfort: pain related to inflammatory process	
3. Poor hygiene related to laziness	Alteration in health maintenance related to feelings of helplessness	This could be related to a number of factors, including feelings of depression, lack of funds, low self-esteem
4. Inability to learn related to learning disability	Self-care deficit related to learning disability	There are a variety of problems that could be related to a learning disability, such as coping, health maintenance, thought processes
5. Needs skin care	Potential impairment of skin integrity related to draining wound	
6. Anger related to diagnosis of cancer	Ineffective coping related to feelings of anger	
7. Alteration in level of consciousness due to transient ischemic attack	Potential for injury related to decreased level of consciousness	
8. Dysfunctional grieving related to death of spouse	Dysfunctional grieving related to denial of loss	
9. Alteration in bodily functions related to vaginal secretions	Alteration in comfort related to infectious process	Depending on the cause of the vaginal secretions, there can be many other problems, including sexual dysfunction, disturbance in self-concept: body image, or self-care deficit: bathing/hygiene
10. Sensory overload related to alteration in thought processes	Alteration in thought processes related to sensory overload	
11. Ineffective breathing patterns related to pneumonia	Ineffective breathing patterns related to infectious process	
12. Alteration in temperature caused by infection	Alteration in comfort related to diaphoresis	
13. Alteration in thought processes related to impaired thinking	Alteration in thought processes related to inability to evaluate reality	
14. Potential for injury related to failure of nurses to put up side rails	Potential for injury related to decreased level of consciousness/immobility	

4–3 TEST YOURSELF

FORMULATION OF DIAGNOSES

Helen O'Brien is a 47 year old white female admitted to your unit. Your assessment reveals the following data: vital signs T = 101° F, B/P = 96/70 mm Hg, P = 110 beats/minute, R = 18 breaths/minute (no abnormal breath sounds), height = 5 ft 5 in, weight = 96 lb. Helen's skin is dry and pale with decreased turgor, and she presents an emaciated appearance. She has no obvious decubiti; however, you note reddened areas on her coccyx and elbows.

She has full range of motion but is unable to walk without assistance since she is often weak and dizzy. Helen indicates that she has fallen twice at home; however, there is no evidence of injury. She is alert and oriented but is obviously tense throughout the interview. She moves her hands continuously and changes position frequently. She cries intermittently and is particularly tearful when her husband is mentioned. She states, "I'm not surprised this happened—I knew I'd get sick if I didn't eat more." She indicates that she has been unable to eat or sleep since the death of her husband two months ago. Helen shares that she is extremely lonely and feels worried and helpless most of the time.

Lab data reveal
   CBC: decreased Hgb and RBC, increased hematocrit
   Urinalysis: concentrated dark amber urine with increased specific gravity, urine culture negative
   Chest x-ray and EKG: normal

How many diagnoses can you identify after reading the case of Mrs. O'Brien?

Nursing Diagnoses

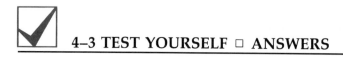

4–3 TEST YOURSELF □ ANSWERS

1. Alteration in nutrition (less than body requirements) related to decreased caloric intake
2. Ineffective coping related to feelings of loneliness and helplessness
3. Potential for injury related to decreased mobility and generalized weakness
4. Sleep pattern disturbance related to grieving
5. Potential impairment in skin integrity related to decreased mobility, impaired nutrition, and decreased hydration

Remember: These are only some of the possibilities. Further assessment will validate your findings.

Reference

Price M. Nursing diagnosis: making a concept come alive. American Journal of Nursing, 668–671, April 1980.

Bibliography

Mundinger M and Jauron G. Developing a nursing diagnosis. Nursing Outlook 23(2):94–98, 1975.

5

Planning— Priority-Setting and Developing Outcomes

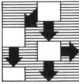

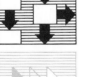

Planning involves the development of strategies designed to prevent, minimize, or correct the problems identified in the nursing diagnosis. This phase begins after the formulation of the diagnostic statement and concludes with the actual documentation of the plan of care.

During the planning phase, outcomes and nursing orders are developed. The outcomes indicate what the client will be able to do as a result of the nursing interventions. The nursing orders describe how the nurse can assist the client to achieve the outcomes.

The planning component of the nursing process consists of four stages:

1. Setting priorities
2. Developing outcomes
3. Developing nursing orders
4. Documentation

This chapter will address the first two stages— priority-setting and developing outcomes.

STAGE 1—SETTING PRIORITIES

A thorough nursing assessment may identify many actual or potential responses that require nursing intervention, as shown in Chapter 4. The development of a plan

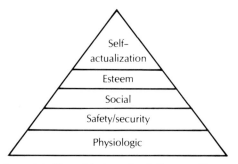

Figure 5-1 □ Maslow's model. (From Maslow, A.: A theory of human motivation. Psychol Rev 50:370, 1943.)

incorporating all of these may be unrealistic or unmanageable. Therefore, a system must be established to determine which diagnosis or diagnoses will be addressed first. One such mechanism is the human needs hierarchy.

Maslow's Hierarchy

Abraham Maslow (1943) described human needs on five levels—physiological, safety or security, social, esteem, and self-actualization (Figure 5–1). He suggested that the client progresses up the hierarchy

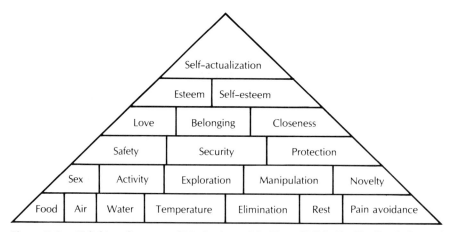

Figure 5-2 □ Kalish's refinement of Maslow's model. (From Kalish, R.: The Psychology of Human Behavior. 5th ed. Copyright 1983, 1977, 1973, 1970, 1966 by Wadsworth, Inc. Reprinted by permission of Brooks/Cole Publishing Co., Monterey, Calif.)

when attempting to satisfy needs. In other words, physiological needs are generally of greater priority to the client than the others. Therefore, when these basic needs are unsatisfied, the client may be unwilling or unable to deal with higher level needs.

Kalish's Hierarchy

Richard Kalish further refined Maslow's system by dividing physiological needs into survival needs and stimulation needs (Figure 5–2). This division is particularly useful in assisting the nurse to prioritize client needs.

Physiological

Survival Needs

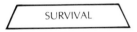

Kalish identified survival needs as those for food, air, water, manageable temperature, elimination, rest, and pain avoidance. When a deficit occurs in any of these areas, the client tends to utilize all available resources to satisfy that particular need. Only then is it possible to be concerned about higher level needs, such as security or esteem.

For this reason, the confused client with an oxygen (air) deficit may continuously climb out of bed to open the window in a hospital room. The basic need for oxygen supersedes concerns about safety. Likewise, the individual who has not slept for three days because of anxiety may not be able to focus on preoperative teaching, even though such information is particularly important to safety in the postoperative period.

Examples of survival needs in nursing diagnostic statements include

Food	Alteration in nutrition: less than body requirements related to anorexia
Air	Impaired gas exchange related to retained secretions
Water	Fluid volume deficit related to persistent vomiting
Temperature	Alteration in comfort related to persistent temperature elevation
Elimination	Alteration in bowel elimination: diarrhea related to effects of antibiotic therapy

Rest   Sleep pattern disturbance related to excessive noise

Pain   Alteration in comfort: pain related to muscle spasms

Stimulation Needs

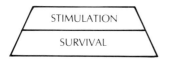

Kalish suggests that stimulation needs include those related to sex, activity, exploration, manipulation, and novelty. When survival needs are met, the client will attempt to satisfy stimulation needs before moving up the hierarchy. For this reason, the younger client who is hospitalized for a prolonged period of time in a psychiatric setting may be unable to focus on therapy when strong sexual urges remain unsatisfied. Similarly, the client who is required to maintain prolonged bedrest at home may require frequent diversionary activities to suppress the desire to get out of bed.

Examples of stimulation needs in nursing diagnostic statements include

Sex   Sexual dysfunction related to discomfort secondary to decreased vaginal secretions

Activity   Diversional activity deficit related to effects of hospitalization

Exploration   Impaired physical mobility related to right-sided weakness

Manipulation   Self-care deficit related to early morning pain secondary to inflammatory process

Novelty   Alteration in sensory perception related to stimulus deprivation secondary to isolation

Case Study

Mr. Ted Alexander, a 50 year old white divorced salesman from Las Vegas, was on a business trip to Atlantic City when he developed pain in the right lower abdominal quadrant. He took Alka-Seltzer with little relief, and the pain persisted for the next two days. He was busy with appointments during the day and evening and was able to ignore the pain. He ate very little and took two sleeping pills at night. On the afternoon of the third day, the pain became much more intense, and when it continued for several hours and he began to vomit repeatedly, he went to the emergency department.

Physical examination and laboratory data at this time revealed an alert, well-groomed male with generalized abdominal tenderness, rigidity of the abdominal wall, presence of a palpable mass in the right inguinal area, absent bowel sounds, and a WBC of 20,000/mm^3 (normal = 5000–9000/mm^3). The diagnosis of ruptured appendix was made. He was admitted to the hospital for initial medical management, with surgery anticipated at a later date.

Your examination of the patient reveals the following: B/P = 140/80 mm Hg, P = 116 beats/minute, R = 26 breaths/minute, T = 101.2°F. The patient indicates that he is 6 ft, 2 in tall and weighs 196 lb. He is alert and oriented and states, "My gut is killing me." His skin is warm to the touch and slightly diaphoretic. The patient states that he had been a heavy drinker for 15 years and was admitted to the hospital with cirrhosis two years ago by his family doctor, Dr. Martland, but has never had surgery. He denies drinking for the past two years but smokes two packs of cigarettes daily.

Mr. Alexander is tense throughout your conversation but shares a number of concerns with you, including his separation from his two teenage children who live with him. He is also anxious about being cared for by an unfamiliar physician. The ED nurse indicates that he wears contact lenses and is concerned because he has left his case and supplies as well as his glasses in his hotel. He gives you $750.00 in cash and traveler's checks to deposit in the hospital safe. He has a partial lower plate of dentures and caps on his four front teeth. Further inquiry reveals that the patient prefers a low-fat diet, occasionally uses laxatives, and has had several occurrences of urinary urgency and nocturia in the last six months.

The physician states that his treatment plan includes gastric suction, antibiotics, and IV fluid therapy with electrolytes and vitamins until the patient is stabilized enough for exploratory surgery. Mr. Alexander agrees to this plan but is concerned about his job demands and wonders how he will deal with "getting back home when all of this is over."

In this example, the primary physiological need is pain avoidance (comfort). The client who experiences pain is frequently unable to deal with higher level concerns. Note that the client verbalized this need in very concrete terms ("My gut is killing me") early in the interview process. This is frequently the case, since the physiological need is the most important reason for the client's visit to the physician's office or to the hospital. Nursing diagnosis: "alteration in comfort: acute abdominal pain related to inflammatory process."

Safety

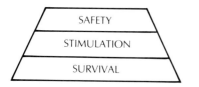

The next level in the hierarchy is the need for safety, security, and protection. These become of particular concern to the client when physiological needs have been satisfied. Safety needs are particularly evident in the elderly or very young when they are placed in an unfamiliar environment. Children frequently require the presence of a favorite toy or blanket for security. The elderly client may be at risk for falls, bruises, and the like while trying to adapt to the strangeness of a nursing home environment.

Some examples of diagnostic statements incorporating safety needs include

Security	Impaired home maintenance management related to insufficient finances
Safety	Potential for injury related to lack of awareness of environmental hazards
Protection	Potential for violence: self-directed related to feelings of hopelessness

Mr. Alexander's concern about being managed by an unfamiliar physician reflects a security need. He has verbalized confidence in his family physician who is 3000 miles away but faces major surgery by a surgeon who is basically unknown to him. Additionally, Mr. Alexander has never had surgery and may be concerned about his safety during the surgical experience. Nursing diagnosis: "potential for ineffective individual coping related to separation from support systems;" "possible knowledge deficit related to surgical experience."

Love and Belonging

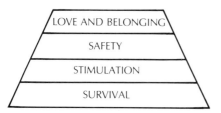

Maslow's social needs are described by Kalish as the necessity for love and a sense of belonging or closeness. These needs relect a person's ability to affiliate or interact with others in the environment and are met through involvement with family, friends, and coworkers. The nurse frequently identifies social deficits in clients requiring prolonged hospitalization, those isolated for protection or because of infection, and those placed in such areas as critical care units, where visiting privileges may be restricted.

Examples of nursing diagnoses reflecting love and belonging needs include

Love	Alteration in parenting related to impaired maternal-infant bonding
Belonging	Alterations in family processes related to ill family member
Closeness	Social isolation related to prolonged hospitalization

Mr. Alexander has verbalized his concern about being separated from his children during hospitalization. This reflects his parental role and the need for interaction with his children. Fulfillment of this need may be particularly difficult because of the children's location. Nursing diagnosis: "potential alteration in parenting related to separation from children."

Esteem

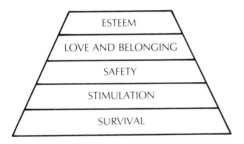

The need for the respect of oneself and others is reflected in this level of the hierarchy. The individual strives for recognition, usefulness, independence, dignity, and freedom. The client's position in the health care system frequently leads to deficits in these areas. Clients may unnecessarily surrender responsibility for elements of daily care to the nurse. Examples might include those who expect the nurse to pour their water, comb their hair, or shave them because they are in a hospital when, in fact, they are capable of self-care.

Examples of nursing diagnoses reflecting esteem needs include "powerlessness related to hospitalization"; "dysfunctional grieving related to alteration in body image secondary to mastectomy"; "disturbance in self-concept: personal identity related to peer pressure."

In Mr. Alexander's case, the need for esteem is demonstrated by his concern about his job demands. Nursing diagnosis: "potential alteration in self-concept: self-esteem related to fear of prolonged disability."

Self-Actualization

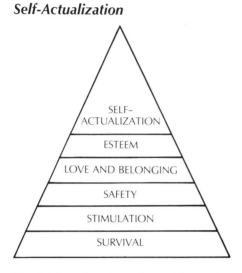

The highest level need is self-actualization, or the need "to make the most of your physical, mental, emotional and social competencies in order to feel that you are being the sort of person you wish to be" (Kalish, 1983). Clients wish to function according to a lifestyle that utilizes their individual knowledge, talents, and skills. Clients in a hospital setting are frequently not concerned with self-actualization needs, since they are preoccupied with fulfilling lower level needs. However, clients may demonstrate concerns about their ability to achieve self-actualization as a result of changes that may have occurred during hospitalization. Nurses who work with clients in other settings, such as their homes, physician's offices, and health maintenance organizations, may see clients who are focusing on self-fulfillment. This is possible because their needs for survival, stimulation, and safety are being satisfied. Therefore, they are able to focus on esteem and self-actualization.

Examples of nursing diagnoses that relate to self-actualization include "alteration in thought processes related to effects of alcohol consumption"; "impaired verbal communication related to expressive aphasia"; "potential for violence related to inability to control behavior"; "family coping: potential for growth related to adequate support systems."

Mr. Alexander has verbalized concern about the effects of the impending surgery on his role as salesman. This reflects a need for self-actualization. Nursing diagnosis: "potential ineffective individual coping related to possible role changes."

Maslow's hierarchy provides a constructive resource for the nurse to utilize in setting priorities. Kalish's expansion of Maslow's model assists the nurse in differentiating more clearly between levels of physiological needs. Ordinarily, clients progress up the hierarchy of needs. For example, they attempt to satisfy survival needs before focusing on security or esteem. However, it is important to note that clients may have unsatisfied needs on more than one level at the same time. Lower level needs do not have to be completely resolved before the client begins to address higher level needs.

Example. Victor Klein, a 48 year old man, is admitted to the hospital with a diagnosis of pneumonia. He exhibits an elevated temperature and is dehydrated. He verbalizes concern about his disabled wife who is confined in bed at home. Additionally, he is self-employed.

In this example, the client has simultaneous survival, security, and love or belonging needs. Mr. Klein's immediate concerns relate to his temperature and fluid problems (survival needs). However, these do not have to be completely resolved before he begins to develop strategies to deal with his anxieties about his job (security) and his disabled wife (love and belonging).

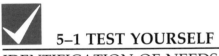 **5–1 TEST YOURSELF**

IDENTIFICATION OF NEEDS

Utilizing Maslow's Hierarchy, identify the type of need being addressed in each of the following nursing diagnoses.

Nursing Diagnosis   **Need**
1. Potential for violence: directed at others, related to hallucinations
2. Disturbance in self-concept: role performance, related to chronic pain
3. Ineffective family coping: disabling, related to marital discord
4. Sleep pattern disturbance related to sensory overload
5. Diversional activity deficit related to long-term confinement
6. Spiritual distress related to inability to practice spiritual rituals
7. Knowledge deficit related to signs of hypoglycemia
8. Disturbance in self-concept: self-esteem, related to obesity
9. Social isolation related to lack of transportation

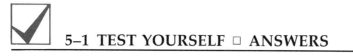

5–1 TEST YOURSELF □ ANSWERS

Nursing Diagnosis	Need
1. Potential for violence: directed at others, related to hallucinations	Safety/security
2. Disturbance in self-concept: role performance, related to chronic pain	Esteem
3. Ineffective family coping: disabling, related to marital discord	Love and belonging
4. Sleep pattern disturbance related to sensory overload	Physiological (survival)
5. Diversional activity deficit related to long-term confinement	Physiological (stimulation)
6. Spiritual distress related to inability to practice spiritual rituals	Self-actualization
7. Knowledge deficit related to signs of hypoglycemia	Safety/security
8. Disturbance in self-concept: self-esteem, related to obesity	Esteem
9. Social isolation related to lack of transportation	Love and belonging

STAGE 2—WRITING OUTCOMES

Nursing diagnostic statements identify actual or potential responses that are considered to be problems for the client. This implies that alternative responses are required or preferred. For example, the nursing diagnosis "alteration in nutrition: less than body requirements, related to chewing difficulties" indicates that the nutritional status of the patient is less than optimal. This diagnosis indicates that improved nutrition is required. Similarly, the nursing diagnosis "potential impairment of skin integrity related to irritating stomal drainage" suggests that the client is at risk for skin breakdown and requires nursing intervention or assistance to prevent its occurrence.

Outcomes should reflect the first half of the diagnostic statement by identifying alternative healthful responses that are desirable for the client. Outcomes also help to define specific behaviors that demonstrate that the problem has been corrected, minimized, or prevented. The outcomes identified below demonstrate alternative behaviors.

Diagnosis	Outcome
Alteration in nutrition (less than body requirements) related to chewing difficulties (broken dentures)	Consumes 1800 calories of puréed and liquid foods each 24 hours

| Potential impairment of skin integrity related to irritating stomal drainage | Applies ostomy pouch with skin barrier every 72 hours |

Although development of outcomes is considered to be an element of the planning process, it also provides a blueprint for the evaluation component. Concise, measurable outcomes that are also reasonable allow the nurse and client to evaluate the client's progress toward the desired outcome. In the first example above, the outcome not only identifies the desirable limits of caloric intake for this client but also specifies that this intake be accomplished within each 24 hour period. The second example describes the activity required to prevent skin breakdown and also suggests a time-frame that is appropriate for the use of skin barriers.

Outcomes are also referred to as goals or behavioral objectives. Regardless of what they are called, their purpose is the same. They are written in a specific fashion to make it possible to evaluate the effectiveness of the nursing interventions.

Guidelines

The rules that guide the formulation of outcomes are based on the premise that outcomes should be easily understandable. A clearly written outcome enhances communication and continuity of care. Nursing personnel who use the nursing care plan should be able to read an outcome and know what it means.

The following rules serve as guidelines for writing understandable outcomes.

1. Outcomes Should Be Client-Centered

Outcomes are written to focus on the behavior of the client. The outcome should address what the client will do and when and to what extent it will be accomplished.

Consider the case of an 82 year old woman who falls and fractures her hip. One of her nursing diagnoses would be "potential impairment of skin integrity related to decreased mobility." The outcome should be written as "throughout hospitalization no evidence of skin breakdown over bony prominences." This clearly identifies the criterion that will be used to evaluate whether or not the skin integrity in this client has been maintained.

2. Outcomes Should be Clear and Concise

Ambiguous or abstract wording should be avoided since it will serve to confuse rather than help the staff caring for a client. Use simple terms and standard terminology. One inventive nurse wrote an outcome as "CDBPD independently q2h." Since these abbreviations were unfamiliar to the rest of the nursing staff, their presence in an outcome resulted in confusion. When this was translated into "cough and deep breath and postural drainage independently q2h," the staff was able to understand the outcome.

The outcome should have as few words as possible yet still be clear. Long, involved outcomes can frequently be stated in fewer words. Compare the following two outcomes. Which meets the criteria of being clear and concise?

The client will discuss expectations of this hospitalization and previous hospital admissions and will discuss impending surgery with a basic knowledge of pre- and post-op care

Prior to surgery, discusses expectations of hospitalization and surgery

When writing outcomes, it is possible to eliminate the words "the client will. . ." at the beginning. It should be obvious from the way the outcome is stated that it is referring to the behaviors the client will exhibit. An exception to this rule would occur if the outcome were to address a family member's behavior instead of or along with the client's behavior. On pediatric units, outcomes are frequently written that involve the parents of the ill child. For example, an outcome could be "Manuel's mother will verbalize her feelings and ask for help when needed."

Outcomes that address the behavior of the client and family or significant other arise when a client and family are expected to demonstrate certain knowledge or skills as a result of teaching. The following outcome illustrates this concept: "by the end of the home visit, client and daughter will describe symptoms of insulin pump malfunction."

3. Outcomes Should Be Observable and Measurable

Previously it was stated that the outcome should address what the client will do, when it will be accomplished, and to what extent. Observable and measurable outcomes include the "what" and "to what extent."

Compare "appreciates the importance of adhering to 1800 calorie

ADA diet" with "adheres to 1800 calorie ADA diet" or "describes importance of adhering to 1800 calorie ADA diet." It is impossible to evaluate
someone's appreciation of the importance of an activity. The client's
recognition and acceptance of the importance of the behavior can be
measured by statements or responses.

When outcomes are measurable, observations can be made to determine whether they have been achieved. Compare "drinks adequate
amounts of fluid" with "drinks 1000 ml in 24 hours." The latter outcome
is observable and measurable.

Sometimes nurses attempt to write an outcome that is too vague, as
in "knows about condition (angina)." This broad outcome needs to be
broken down into separate outcomes. These might include the causes of
angina, management of the pain, and knowledge of preventive health
practices. These outcomes should be written so that they are observable
by using such words as "describes," "identifies," and "lists."

☐ "Lists the causes of angina"
☐ "Identifies steps to alleviate pain"
☐ "Describes three activities that reduce anginal episodes"

4. Outcomes Should Be Time-Limited

The time for achievement of the outcome should be stated. Examples of
these statements include "by the time of discharge," "throughout hospitalization," "by the end of the teaching session," and "within 48 hours."
These suggest the time-frame for evaluating the achievement of each
outcome.

5. Outcomes Should Be Realistic

The outcomes should be achievable with the resources of the client,
nursing staff, and agency. The client's readiness to achieve the outcomes
will be affected by many factors, including finances, level of intelligence,
and emotional and physical condition.

Example. A diabetic hindered by a low income might have a great deal of
difficulty in purchasing a home glucose monitoring system. Therefore, it
may be unrealistic to write an outcome and set up a teaching plan
encouraging the use of this system.

The strengths and weaknesses of the nursing staff should be considered when formulating outcomes. Factors to evaluate include the nurses' level of knowledge, autonomy, and availability.

Example. A woman who is pregnant with triplets is admitted to an obstetrical unit. None of the nurses working in the department has cared for a similar patient. The perinatal clinical specialist has knowledge of the special care required in this situation. The specialist provides the information and assists the staff to formulate realistic client outcomes.

Finally, the resources of the agency must be considered when formulating outcomes. Factors to take into account include the availability of equipment, facilities, and nonnursing personnel.

Examples

The Ideal	Reality
"Spends four hours a day in a wheelchair."	There are two wheelchairs on a 30 bed unit.
"Showers every day by 9:00 A.M."	There are six clients who need to use the same shower by 9:00 A.M.

Clearly the outcomes must be realistic for the setting in which they are written. Additionally, the nursing staff must be flexible enough to modify unrealistic or unachievable outcomes.

6. Outcomes Should Be Determined by the Client and Nurse Together

During the initial assessment, the nurse begins involving the client in the planning of care. In the interview, the nurse learns about what the client sees as the primary health problem. This leads to the formulation of nursing diagnoses. The client and nurse discuss the outcomes and plan of care to validate them. In this discussion, they will communicate their expectations. Together they will have an opportunity to modify any unrealistic outcomes. The inclusion of the client as an active participant in the plan of care will help ensure the achievement of the outcomes.

Example. Sophie Lean is a 68 year old diabetic who is admitted with diabetic retinopathy and gangrene of the left foot. She lives with her sister, Florence. Since Sophie has limited vision, Florence assists with her hygiene. During the interview, Florence asks the nurse to review the care of Sophie's feet. The nurse says, "By the time Sophie leaves the hospital, we will review how to wash and dry her feet, the signs of an infection, and what to do if you find an infection. How does this sound?" Florence says, "Yes, that's what I want."

During this conversation the nurse has set outcomes and validated them with Florence. By the time of discharge, the client's sister will

☐ Demonstrate proper foot care
☐ Describe signs of infection
☐ State the course of action to follow if infection occurs

One of the consequences of not validating outcomes with a client may be the client's refusal to participate in the plan of care. This may occur if the client feels the outcomes are impossible to achieve or are opposed to the client's values.

Example. Reverend Johnson had a repair of a ventral hernia eight hours ago. The nurse on the surgical floor offers him an injection of pain medication. He refuses, saying he can do without it. The nurse notes that he is diaphoretic, pale, and lying in a rigid position. On three more occasions during the shift the nurse offers him pain medication, which is refused. The nurse begins to feel frustrated because the medication is being rejected.

Compare

The nurse's desired outcome for Reverend Johnson: asks for pain medication when needed; expresses relief after receiving medication

Reverend Johnson's goal for himself: get through this hospitalization without having to take a shot

The nurse and the client are now in a conflict situation and must use strategies to resolve the disagreement and to formulate an outcome that is acceptable to both of them. By exploring his reasons for refusal of the injection and offering acceptable pain management techniques, the nurse will be involving him in the decision-making about his care. Alternate approaches might include oral analgesics, relaxation or distraction techniques, or transcutaneous electrical nerve stimulation (TENS).

Manifestations of Human Responses

Outcomes can be written to cover a number of human responses, including appearance and functioning of the body, symptoms, knowledge, skills, and emotions.

Appearance and Functioning of the Body

This category includes a number of observable manifestations. The following outcome written for a woman with a fractured hip fits into this category: "Throughout hospitalization no evidence of skin breakdown over bony prominences." This is a readily observable outcome that relates to the appearance of her skin.

Other examples

Nursing Diagnoses for Post-op Clients	Outcomes
Alteration in bowel elimination related to decreased peristalsis and change in diet	Within 48 hours after surgery: bowel sounds present; expels flatus or BM; abdomen is soft By time of discharge, returns to normal elimination pattern
Potential impaired gas exchange related to incisional pain	Lung sounds clear each shift; demonstrates equal expansion of chest wall during inspiration
Potential impairment of skin integrity related to infection	At time of discharge, no evidence of infection at suture line

The above outcomes all relate to the appearance or functioning of the client's body. It is important to note that a nursing diagnosis may be accompanied by more than one outcome. Sometimes several outcomes are needed to evaluate whether the actual problem has been changed or the potential problem prevented.

Specific Symptoms

Outcomes may be written to address the reduction or alleviation of symptoms that are interfering with the client's health status. Examples of symptoms include nausea, vomiting, diarrhea, constipation, burning sensation while urinating, frequent urination, pain, stiffness, weakness, and so on. The nurse identifies the symptoms, writes outcomes addressing them, and plans nursing interventions to alleviate them.

Nursing Diagnoses	Outcomes
Alteration in comfort: pain related to decreased mobility	Asks for pain medication when needed; expresses relief after initiation of comfort measures

Nursing Diagnoses	Outcomes
Alteration in nutrition: less than body requirements related to persistent vomiting and dehydration	Free of vomiting within one hour of administration of antiemetics; drinks 1000 ml of fluid in 24 hours

Knowledge

Outcomes may be formulated that involve the recall of information taught to the client. To determine whether the material has been mastered, the client should be asked to list, describe, state, define, or otherwise demonstrate knowledge of some concrete pieces of information.

Nursing Diagnosis	Outcomes
Potential alteration in health maintenance related to lack of knowledge about diabetes	By end of first teaching session: defines diabetes; explains relationship between diet, insulin, and activity.

Psychomotor Skills

Psychomotor skills can be the subject of outcomes. Examples include

□ Injection of medications
□ Transfer from bed to wheelchair
□ Catheterizing self or others
□ Counting a pulse
□ Performing CPR on a mannequin
□ Inserting intravenous catheters
□ Testing urine or blood for glucose

The outcomes that are written for psychomotor skills identify what the client should be able to do as a result of the teaching plan.

Nursing Diagnoses	Outcomes
Potential for alteration in health maintenance related to lack of knowledge about diabetes	By the end of the second teaching session: demonstrates proper technique for foot care; tests urine for glucose and acetone
Potential alteration in parenting related to lack of knowledge of newborn care and breast feeding	By the time of discharge: feeds and diapers newborn; demonstrates effective breast-feeding techniques

Emotional Status

Outcomes may be written about the emotional status of the client. These outcomes address how the client or family is responding to a stressful event. This may be an illness, family disruption, or a maturational crisis. After assessing the emotional response, the nurse develops an outcome identifying the desired behavior that should result from nursing intervention.

Nursing Diagnoses	Outcomes
Ineffective parental coping related to lack of support systems	Throughout hospitalization, Manuel's mother will identify available resources
Disturbance in self-concept: self-esteem related to change in body image secondary to mastectomy	Prior to discharge: verbalizes feelings about loss of breast; initiates positive interactions with staff, visitors, and roommate

SUMMARY

Outcomes should be client-centered, clear, concise, observable, measurable, time-limited, realistic, and determined by the client and nurse together. The areas in which outcomes may be written include appearance and functioning of the body, specific symptoms, knowledge, psychomotor skills, and emotional status. Consideration of these factors will enable the nurse to formulate outcomes that are useful and easily evaluated.

![checkmark] **5–2 TEST YOURSELF**

IDENTIFICATION OF CORRECTLY AND INCORRECTLY WRITTEN OUTCOMES

Following is a list of outcomes. Decide whether each outcome is correctly or incorrectly written. If incorrectly stated, identify, by number, the rule(s) violated from the list below.

Rules

1. Client-centered
2. Clear and concise
3. Observable and measurable
4. Time-limited
5. Realistic
6. Determined by client and nurse together

	Correct	Incorrect	Rule(s)
1. Dies with dignity			
2. By the time of discharge, transfers safely from bed to wheelchair			
3. After surgery, verbalizes feelings about loss of childbearing ability			
4. Injects self with insulin			
5. Prevent accidents			
6. Temperature within normal limits 24 hours after surgery			
7. Client will be free of frequency and urgency in urination, cloudy, foul-smelling urine, dysuria, and temperature elevation			
8. By the time of discharge, verbalizes complete acceptance of loss of breast			
9. Before surgery, verbalizes fears regarding outcome of surgery			
10. Client and family (Jehovah's Witnesses) will sign permit for blood transfusion			
11. Client will receive support from staff			
12. Loses two lb per week until achieves weight of 110 lb			

5–2 TEST YOURSELF □ ANSWERS

Rules
1. Client-centered
2. Clear and concise
3. Observable and measurable
4. Time-limited
5. Realistic
6. Determined by client and nurse together

	Correct	Incorrect	Rule(s)
1. Dies with dignity		✔	3
2. By the time of discharge, transfers safely from bed to wheelchair	✔		
3. After surgery, verbalizes feelings about loss of childbearing ability	✔		
4. Injects self with insulin		✔	3, 4
5. Prevent accidents		✔	1
6. Temperature within normal limits 24 hours after surgery	✔		
7. Client will be free of frequency and urgency in urination, cloudy, foul-smelling urine, dysuria, and temperature elevation		✔	2, 4
8. By the time of discharge, verbalizes complete acceptance of loss of breast		✔	5
9. Before surgery, verbalizes fears regarding outcome of surgery	✔		
10. Client and family (Jehovah's Witnesses) will sign permit for blood transfusion		✔	6
11. Client will receive support from staff		✔	1, 3, 4
12. Loses two lb a week until achieves weight of 110 lb	✔		

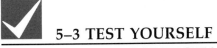

5–3 TEST YOURSELF

REVISION OF INCORRECTLY WRITTEN OUTCOMES

The outcomes that were incorrectly written are listed below. A nursing diagnosis has been defined for each outcome to assist you in formulating a new outcome. Revise each outcome so that it is correctly stated.

Nursing Diagnosis	Outcome	Revised Outcome
1. Anticipatory grieving related to awareness of impending death	Dies with dignity	
2. Alteration in health maintenance related to lack of knowledge about insulin injections	Injects self with insulin	
3. Potential for injury related to decreased level of consciousness	Prevent accidents	
4. Potential alteration in urinary elimination related to infection secondary to catheterization	Client will be free of frequency and urgency in urination, cloudy, foul-smelling urine, dysuria, and temperature elevation	
5. Disturbance in self-concept: body image related to fear of rejection secondary to mastectomy	By the time of discharge, verbalizes complete acceptance of loss of breast	
6. Noncompliance (signing blood permit) related to religious beliefs (Jehovah's Witness)	Client and family (Jehovah's Witnesses) will sign permit for blood transfusion	
7. Ineffective individual coping related to feelings of hopelessness	Client will receive support from staff	

5-3 TEST YOURSELF □ ANSWERS

The following are suggested answers for the preceding exercise. Keep in mind that there is more than one way to revise an outcome.

Nursing Diagnosis	Outcome	Revised Outcome	Comments
1. Anticipatory grieving related to awareness of impending death	Dies with dignity	Prior to death, verbalizes acceptance of death	The way this goal is written depends on the client's stage of acceptance of death (according to Kubler-Ross and others)
2. Alteration in health maintenance related to lack of knowledge about insulin injections	Injects self with insulin	By the end of teaching session, uses sterile technique to inject self with insulin	
3. Potential for injury related to decreased level of consciousness	Prevent accidents	Throughout hospitalization, experiences no injuries or accidents	
4. Potential alteration in urinary elimination related to infection secondary to catheterization	Client will be free of frequency and urgency in urination, cloudy, foul-smelling urine, dysuria, and temperature elevation	Throughout hospitalization, no evidence of urinary tract infection	Since the symptoms of urinary tract infections are widely known, it is not necessary to spell them out
5. Disturbance in self-concept: body image related to fear of rejection secondary to mastectomy	By the time of discharge, verbalizes complete acceptance of loss of breast	By the time of discharge, verbalizes feelings about loss of breast	
6. Noncompliance (signing blood permit) related to religious beliefs (Jehovah's Witness)	Client and family (Jehovah's Witnesses) will sign permit for blood transfusion	Client and family verbalize awareness of hazards of refusing blood	This outcome could be written many different ways depending on the gravity of the situation and the strength of the client's convictions
7. Ineffective individual coping related to feelings of hopelessness	Client will receive support from staff	Prior to discharge, identifies support systems for coping with illness	Putting the words "the client will" before a nurse-centered goal does not make it a patient-centered goal

✓ 5–4 TEST YOURSELF

DEVELOPMENT OF OUTCOMES FROM A CASE STUDY

Helen O'Brien is a 47 year old white female admitted to your unit. Your assessment reveals the following vital signs: T = 101° F, B/P = 96/70 mm Hg, P = 110 beats/minute, R = 18 breaths/minute (no abnormal breath sounds), height = 5 ft 5 in, weight = 96 lb. Helen's skin is dry and pale with decreased turgor, and she has an emaciated appearance. She has no obvious decubiti; however, you note reddened areas on her coccyx and elbows.

She has full range of motion but is unable to walk without assistance, since she is often weak and dizzy. Helen indicates that she has fallen twice at home; however, there is no evidence of injury. She is alert and oriented but is obviously tense throughout the interview. She moves her hands continuously and changes position frequently. She cries intermittently and is particularly tearful when her husband is mentioned. She states, "I'm not surprised this happened—I knew I'd get sick if I didn't eat more." She indicates that she has been unable to eat or sleep since the death of her husband two months ago. Helen shares that she is extremely lonely and feels worried and helpless most of the time.

Lab data reveal:
> CBC: decreased Hgb and RBC, increased hematocrit
> Urinalysis: concentrated dark amber urine with increased
> specific gravity; urine culture negative
> Chest x-ray and EKG: normal

For each nursing diagnosis, formulate an outcome using the guidelines previously identified.

Nursing Diagnoses

Outcomes

1. Alteration in nutrition: less than body requirements related to decreased caloric intake
2. Ineffective individual coping related to feelings of loneliness and helplessness
3. Potential for injury related to dizziness and weakness
4. Sleep pattern disturbance related to insomnia secondary to grieving
5. Potential impairment of skin integrity related to decreased nutrition and hydration

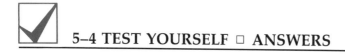

5-4 TEST YOURSELF □ ANSWERS

Nursing Diagnoses	Outcomes
1. Alteration in nutrition (less than body requirements) related to decreased caloric intake	Consumes 2000 calories daily
2. Ineffective individual coping related to feelings of loneliness and helplessness	By the time of discharge, identifies available support systems
3. Potential for injury related to dizziness and weakness	Calls for assistance before ambulating; throughout hospitalization, no evidence of injury
4. Sleep pattern disturbance related to insomnia secondary to grieving	Sleeps four hours each night without interruption
5. Potential impairment of skin integrity related to decreased nutrition and hydration	Throughout hospitalization, no evidence of skin breakdown; drinks 2500 ml of fluid daily

References

Kalish R. The Psychology of Human Behavior. 5th ed. Monterey, California: Brooks/Cole Publishing Company, 1983.

Maslow A. A theory of human motivation. Psychol Rev 50:370, 1943.

Bibliography

Christensen P. Goals and objectives. In Griffith J and Christensen P: Nursing Process. St. Louis: CV Mosby, 1982.

Inzer F and Aspinall M. Evaluating patient outcomes. Nursing Outlook 178–181, March 1981.

Kozier B and Erb G. Fundamentals of Nursing Concepts and Procedures. 1st ed. Menlo Park, California: Addison-Wesley Publishing Company, 1979.

Nussbaum J. Care Planning for Nurses. 2nd ed. Thorofare, NJ: Charles B. Slack, 1981.

Smith D. Writing objectives as a nursing practice skill. In Lamonica E. Nursing Process. Menlo Park, California: Addison-Wesley Publishing Company, 1979.

Snyder P. Goal setting. Supervisor Nurse 61–64, September 1978.

6

Planning—Nursing Orders and Documentation

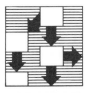

The stages of the planning phase of the nursing process are (1) setting priorities, (2) developing outcomes, (3) designing nursing orders, and (4) documentation. The first two stages were addressed in the previous chapter. Once priorities have been established and outcomes developed, the next stages of planning begin.

The third stage involves writing nursing orders, which describe how the nurse will assist the client to achieve the proposed outcomes. These orders are based on (1) the information obtained during the assessment interview and (2) the nurse's subsequent interactions with the client and family. The final phase—documentation—involves communicating the written plan of care to other members of the nursing staff. This chapter will address these last two stages of the planning phase—developing nursing orders and documenting the plan of care.

STAGE III—NURSING ORDERS

Definition

Nursing orders are specific interventions designed to assist the client to achieve outcomes. They are based on the etiology component of the nursing diagnostic statement. Therefore, nursing orders define the activities required to eliminate the factors contributing to the problem.

Example. "Potential for injury related to hazardous home environment." The nursing orders in this case would focus on reducing the environmental hazards in the client's home.

Comparison of Nursing and Medical Orders

Medical or physician's orders usually focus on the activities involved in diagnosing and treating the client's medical condition. These orders are delegated to nurses and other health care personnel. Medical orders often include administration of medications, diagnostic tests, dietary requirements, and treatments.

Nursing orders focus on the activities required to promote, maintain, or restore the client's health. They may be categorized as dependent, interdependent, or independent.

Dependent Orders

Dependent orders relate to the implementation of medical orders. They indicate the manner in which the medical order is to be carried out.

Example. The physician writes an order to weigh a client three times weekly. The nurse clarifies the order as follows: "Weigh Monday, Wednesday, and Friday. Use bedscale."

Example. The physician writes an order for "colostomy care." The nursing orders define colostomy care based on the individual needs of the client. These orders could include

"Perform colostomy care every two days or when appliance is leaking."

"Remove pouch gently, starting at the edges. May use soap and water to loosen adhesive."

"Cleanse peristomal area with soap and water; allow to dry completely."

"Examine skin and stoma for signs and symptoms of irritation."

"Apply skin prep to peristomal area."

"Apply Bongort pouch, size 1¾ in."

"Review each step verbally with client and his wife."

Interdependent Orders

Interdependent nursing orders describe the activities that the nurse carries out in cooperation with other health team members. The orders may involve collaboration with social workers, dieticians, therapists, technicians, and physicians.

Example. Barrett Bleakley is a client who is in renal failure. The medical order states "restrict fluids to 600 ml by mouth plus 720 ml 5% dextrose in .45 sodium chloride solution IV every 24 hours." To define how this will be achieved, the nurse and dietician calculate the amount of fluid Barrett may receive each shift. The nursing orders are as follows.
    1. IV fluids to run at 30 ml/hr (total of 240 ml per shift). Run via IV pump.
    2. PO fluid intake:
        7:30 A.M.–3:30 P.M.—Total of 315 ml po
                           240 ml on dietary trays
                           75 ml for medications
        3:30–11:30 P.M.—Total of 195 ml po
                           120 ml on dietary tray
                           75 ml for medications
        11:30 P.M.–7:30 A.M.—Total of 100 ml po for medications

Independent Orders

Independent nursing orders are the activities that may be performed by the nurse without a direct physician's order. The type of activities that nurses may order independently are defined by nursing diagnoses. They are the responses that nurses are licensed to treat by virtue of their education and experience.

Example. Constance Lance is an 82 year old woman who fell and broke her hip. She says to the nurse, "I am going to have to watch myself when I go home. I don't want to hurt myself again." The nurse writes the following orders:
    "Assist the client to identify potential hazards at home."
    "Notify son of concerns and seek his involvement in correcting hazards."
    "Encourage client to request home hazard survey by the visiting nurse prior to discharge."

Characteristics of Orders

Nursing orders should have certain desirable characteristics. They should
1. Be consistent with the plan of care.
2. Be based on scientific principles.
3. Be individualized to the specific situation.
4. Be used to provide a safe and therapeutic environment.
5. Employ teaching-learning opportunities for the client.
6. Include utilization of appropriate resouces (ANA, 1973).

Consistency

The nursing orders should not be in conflict with the therapeutic approaches of other members of the health team. When nurses and other professionals are working at cross-purposes, confusion and frustration result. It is important that members of various disciplines communicate their goals and define approaches to achieve those goals. Any differences of opinion need to be resolved to promote coordinated care.

Example. Kathy Smith works as an office nurse for a family practice physician. Eric Baker, a nine year old insulin-dependent diabetic, has been receiving insulin for three years. Up to this point, Eric's mother has been responsible for the insulin injections. Kathy believes that Eric, who is very bright, is ready to learn how to inject himself. When Kathy writes her orders to begin teaching, the physician objects. "He's too young to learn how to give himself insulin. I don't want him to be taught that yet."

The physician and the nurse disagree in this situation. It is important that they resolve this conflict to promote a consistent approach to Eric's care.

Scientific Basis

The nursing orders prescribed for an individual client should evolve from sound nursing judgment. A scientific rationale supports the nurse's decisions and forms the foundation for nursing action. This rationale is developed from the nurse's knowledge base, which includes natural and behavioral sciences and the humanities. Each nursing order should be supported by scientific principles. The following examples demonstrate nursing orders and associated scientific principles.

Nursing Order	Scientific Principle
1. Encourage client to identify hazards in his home	1. Elderly clients are at greater risk for injuries and falls
2. Teach client to rotate insulin injection sites	2. Repeated use of the same site may cause fibrosis, scarring, and decreased insulin absorption

3. Increase fluids to 2500 ml daily
   7–3   1300 ml
   3–11   800 ml
   11–7   400 ml
	3. Adequate fluid intake is necessary to maintain normal stool consistency

Although scientific principles are usually not included in the written nursing order, the nurse must have a thorough understanding of the rationale for nursing actions. This allows modification of the nursing order, if necessary, without violating the principles upon which it is based.

Example

Nursing Order	Rationale
Turn q2h and massage bony prominences with lotion	Reduction of pressure and increased circulation decreases the potential for skin breakdown

While turning the client, the nurse notices a reddened area on the right heel and adds an order for a wafer barrier. The rationale is the same.

Apply Duoderm to right heel	Reduction of pressure on the skin surface decreases the potential for skin breakdown

Occasionally the principles may be incorporated into the nursing order for clarification or explanation.

Example. "Encourage client to feed self starting 1/15/86 to promote independence."

Individualization

One purpose of nursing orders is to communicate how one client's care differs from that of another with a similar nursing or medical diagnosis. When developing nursing orders, the nurse chooses approaches that will address the client's specific physical and emotional needs. The following are guidelines that should be used in the development of individualized nursing orders.

1. Focus on the nursing diagnosis and the outcome.
2. Include the input of the client and family in choosing alternatives.
3. Consider client and family strengths and weaknesses.
4. Take into account the urgency and severity of the situation.

Focus on Nursing Diagnosis. The nursing diagnostic statement provides a basis for establishing individualized nursing orders. As explained previously, the nursing diagnosis has two parts—the problem and the etiology. The etiology specifies the origin of the problem and provides direction for specific nursing orders. The nurse's knowledge of the client and the problem directs the formulation of individualized nursing orders.

Example

Dona Vessels is a 17 year old hospitalized following a motorcycle accident. She is in skeletal traction for a fractured left leg.

Betsey Moehlich, an 84 year old, is a resident of a nursing home. She is thin, slightly dehydrated, and is confined in bed.

Nursing diagnosis: "potential alteration in skin integrity related to immobility."

Nursing Orders

Dona	Betsey
1. Apply foam mattress to bed	1. Apply air mattress to bed
2. Massage bony prominences with lotion q4h (10 A.M., 2 P.M., 6 P. M.)	2. Assist client to change position q2h (see turning schedule). Include prone position at least once per shift.
3. Encourage client to use trapeze to change position	3. Massage bony prominences with lotion q4h after turning.

Note that although the nursing diagnosis is the same for both clients, the nursing orders are individualized.

Client Input. After nursing diagnoses are established, outcomes are formulated with the client's input. The involvement of the client in outcome development increases the potential for individualization of nursing orders. After nursing orders are formulated, they are reviewed with the client. This ensures that the planned interventions are understood by and are acceptable and applicable to the individual client. Frequently, clients will participate more actively in their care if their ideas have been solicited.

Example. Ida Gold, an 85 year old woman, was recently discharged from the hospital after a total knee replacement. She is being cared for at home by a private duty nurse. Since Ida prefers to sit in a wheelchair all day, the nurse recognizes the potential for skin breakdown. The private duty nurse shares her concern with Ida and asks for her help in identifying other positions of comfort. Ida agrees to take short walks a few times a day to relieve the pressure on her skin.

Strengths and Weaknesses. When developing individualized nursing orders, the strengths and weaknesses of the client and the family must be considered. The client's assets should be identified and utilized in planning care. Strengths may include motivation, intelligence, a supportive family, education, or economic resources.

Example. Erin Mirabelli is a 22 year old newly diagnosed insulin-dependent diabetic. Erin is a highly motivated and self-disciplined young woman. She worked her way through college and graduated with a degree in biology. She is currently employed as a laboratory technician in industry. She maintains an active schedule, including aerobics and weight lifting.

The nurse practitioner decided to utilize Erin's strengths in planning her education on diabetic management. Erin was provided with self-learning packages on the fundamentals of pathology and management. She was also identified as a good candidate for blood glucose monitoring to determine her blood sugar and subsequent insulin needs.

The client's weaknesses or deficits should also be identified. The absence of motivation, intelligence, family support, economic resources, or education may act as a deterrent to health. Other deficits might include chronic illness, debilitation, depression, social withdrawal, or a language barrier.

In the following situation, the nurse considered the client's physical deficits when planning care.

Example. Roberto Reilly, a 56 year old man with emphysema, is admitted to the hospital following a cerebrovascular accident (CVA). The nursing orders include: "Assist the client to conserve his energy by resting after meals and bathing."

The physician orders physical therapy for Roberto's right-sided weakness. Promptly at 9:00 A.M., just after Roberto finishes breakfast, the physical therapist arrives at his bedside to begin passive range of motion exercises. Roberto looks at the nurse and says "Do I really have to go through this now?" The nurse discusses Roberto's limitations with the therapist and determines a more appropriate time for the therapy.

In this case, the nurse develops a nursing order for rest intervals based on an assessment of Roberto's physical limitations. Additionally, the nurse acts as a client advocate in assisting with the individualization of the physical therapy.

These two examples demonstrate that individualized nursing orders result from the nurse's consideration of the client's strengths and weaknesses when making decisions for care.

Severity and Urgency of Condition. At times, the severity or urgency of the client's problem may influence the nursing order. This occurs when the alteration in health may result in harm to the client or to others.

Example. Michael York, an elderly client, has an adverse reaction to a sleeping medication. He becomes confused and violent when the nurse attempts to reorient him. This situation requires immediate independent intervention. The nurse implements the following individualized nursing orders.

□ Safely protect the client in bed with a jacket restraint
□ Assign a nursing assistant to stay with him until the client is reoriented.
□ Inform the physician of the change in the client's behavior

In the critical care setting, the client's condition may be so severe that participation in planning care may be impossible. Therefore, the nurse functions as the client's advocate and makes decisions based on nursing expertise and scientific principles. The nursing orders in this instance are individualized and based on the severity of the problem.

Provision of a Safe and Therapeutic Environment

When planning nursing orders, the nurse must consider the satisfaction of the client's physical and emotional needs. A safe environment is one in which the client's physiological needs are met and the client is protected from potential injury. A therapeutic environment assists the client in resolving the health problem and satisfying the need for interpersonal relationships.

Safe Environment. As described in Chapter 5, physiological needs—for air, food, rest, water—must be satisfied before higher level needs can be addressed. In a safe environment, these basic needs are provided for by nursing and medical interventions. Examples of nursing orders that assist in the satisfaction of basic needs follow.

□ Provide 2000 ml or clear fluids in 24 hours (food).
□ Assess need for oxygen and provide via mask at 4 liters/minute (air).
□ Encourage client to drink 60 ml prune juice each morning (elimination).
□ Provide 30 minute rest intervals after meals (rest/sleep).

Those clients who are particularly at risk for injury include infants and children and those who are elderly, debilitated, or under anesthesia.

There are numerous nursing actions designed to create a safe environment for these individuals. Common nursing orders include the following.

☐ Side rails up at all times.
☐ Restrain with Posey belt when necessary.
☐ Place bedside table within reach (for client on bedrest).
☐ Monitor client while smoking.
☐ Teach parents to child-proof house.
☐ Instruct the (elderly) client on potential hazards in home.
☐ Teach parent to keep rail of crib up at all times.
☐ Assist the (elderly) client into the tub, checking bath water temperature carefully.
☐ Assess client for adequate oxygenation while intubated q 15 minutes.

Therapeutic Environment. Nursing orders are developed to identify interventions that are effective in the promotion, maintenance, or restoration of health. The orders may consist of treatments, assessment, teaching, consultations, or any other types of interventions likely to be helpful.

Examples

☐ Teach the client foods to avoid while taking anticoagulants.
☐ Assess for the presence of incisional pain; medicate prn.
☐ Consult with social service re: nursing home placement.
☐ Range of motion exercises for legs qid.

The caring environment is therapeutic for the client. The nurse demonstrates concern by the nonverbal components of behavior—tone of voice, touch, and eye contact. The nurse also conveys compassion by such actions as treating the client with respect and courtesy, by listening, and by being helpful.

Nursing orders that help to create a therapeutic environment include the following.

☐ Notify client's son when client returns from recovery room.
☐ Assist the client to identify support groups in the community.
☐ Encourage client to verbalize feelings about loss of spouse.

Teaching-Learning Opportunities

The teaching-learning process for the client includes the acquisition of new knowledge, attitudes, and skills and related changes in behavior. The nursing orders involved in the teaching-learning process include the following.

1. Assess the client's learning needs.
2. Determine the client's readiness to learn.
3. Identify the factors that influence the client's ability to learn.
4. Develop individualized outcomes that are realistic and attainable.
5. Determine strategies to assist the client and family to achieve desired outcomes.
6. Present content in an understandable fashion using appropriate resources.
7. Evaluate the client's progress toward achievement of outcomes.
8. Modify the plan as required.

Assess Learning Needs. Prior to the initiation of a teaching plan, the nurse should gather data to evaluate the client's individual learning needs. Clients should be encouraged to identify the needs they perceive as important. These needs may be evidenced by direct questions, such as "What happens when they do an ultrasound?" "Why can't I eat after midnight when I'm going for surgery tomorrow?" "How do I get dressed with this cast on?"

Learning needs may also be identified by observing the client's condition or behavior. For instance, the visiting nurse notes that the skin around Mr. Conover's stoma is red and excoriated. The nurse questions the client and determines that he has not been using a skin barrier because it is "too expensive." Or the school nurse observes that Maria Brown does not wash her hands before leaving the bathroom. These situations demonstrate indirect identification of client learning needs.

At times, clients may directly identify their learning needs by requesting information to promote, maintain, or restore their health.

Example. Rorie Parrella is a 30 year old who had a biopsy for a benign breast mass. The nurse questions the client regarding her ability to do breast self-examination. The client indicates that she's not sure how to do it but would like to learn.

Here the nurse's intervention will assist the client to maintain her health by early detection of additional masses.

Determine Readiness to Learn. The client must be physically and emotionally prepared for the teaching-learning experience. The nurse should initiate interventions directed to relief of pain, fear, anxiety, or fatigue before attempting to involve the client in learning activities.

Example. Verna MacCarthy is admitted to the hospital with essential hypertension. She indicates that she wants to know more about her disease and what she can do to lower her blood pressure. The nurse goes to Verna's room to begin teaching but finds the client in bed, holding her head and complaining of a severe headache.

In this case, the nurse recognizes that although the client is motivated to learn, the physical discomfort associated with headache may interfere with her ability to concentrate on or absorb the information presented. Therefore, the nurse decides to defer teaching to another time.

Example. Bill Ryder is in the coronary care unit with an acute myocardial infarction (heart attack). The nurse explains the use of monitoring equipment but detects that the client does not retain the information. He repeatedly asks "Am I OK, nurse?"

In this situation, the nurse recognizes that the client is unable to absorb even simple explanations of routines and equipment because he is afraid of dying. Therefore, the nurse will continue to provide brief bits of factual information until the client demonstrates readiness to accept additional information.

Identify Factors Influencing Ability to Learn. There are a number of factors that affect the client's ability to learn, including preexisting knowledge, level of education, age, motivation, state of health, and lifestyle.

Clients' current level of knowledge, including their misconceptions and misinformation, frequently affects their ability to learn. Some knowledge is prerequisite for additional learning. For example, clients who need to change a sterile dressing may encounter great difficulty if they do not know the basics of good hand-washing.

Level of education frequently defines clients' knowledge of health and disease. If the information presented is above that level, the client may be unable to learn. The reverse may also be true. If information is presented at a level significantly below the client's level of education, the client might feel insulted and therefore fail to learn the material.

Age also affects ability to learn. The very young child may have difficulty in grasping concepts unless they are presented in very concrete terms. Some elderly clients may have ingrained ideas or "myths" that affect their ability to accept new changes. Additionally, they may have physiological deficits that interfere with their ability to learn (e.g., vision or hearing problems).

Clients must also be motivated to learn. Generally, they will readily learn whatever is most important to them. This substantiates the need for an accurate assessment of the client's perceived needs. However, not all clients desire information. Some prefer to delegate the responsibility for promoting, maintaining, or restoring their health to family members or health care personnel. Others in a state of denial may refuse to acknowledge the need to learn about their illness. Therefore, it is very difficult for these clients to learn effectively.

The state of health of the client may affect ability to learn. The client with a critical illness, severe debilitation, or sensory-perceptual deficits may be unable to process or absorb information. This may also be the case for clients with terminal disease, since they may lack motivation or ability.

The client's lifestyle may affect ability to learn. This is particularly pertinent when considering low socioeconomic groups and people of certain cultures. The client's learning problem may be associated with deficits in the types of experiences that make learning a desirable outcome. The client may not be stimulated in his or her culture to learn content perceived to be unnecessary or unimportant. Certain personality types—e.g., dependent or irresponsible persons—may also have inherent motivational problems.

Develop Individualized Outcomes. The learning outcomes for each client involve knowledge, attitudes, and skills. For example, the nurse may be required to teach the client who needs an ostomy the following.

☐ How the surgery has altered the gastrointestinal tract (knowledge)
☐ How the ostomy will affect the client's lifestyle (knowledge)
☐ What types of equipment are necessary to manage the ostomy (knowledge)
☐ How to cleanse the stromal area and apply a pouch (skill)
☐ How to irrigate the ostomy (skill)

After acquiring this knowledge and these skills, the client may express confidence (attitude) in the ability to manage this major lifestyle change.

Outcomes must be realistic. The involvement of the client in outcome decisions helps to assure that they will be realistic. Accurate assessment of the client's motivation and abilities is also critical.

Example. Steven Sturgeon is seen in a drug rehabilitation clinic. The nurse develops the following teaching goal: "identifies the effects of prolonged drug abuse at the end of the first teaching session." This outcome is not realistic for Steven, since he is still experiencing the effects of the drugs he is taking. A more realistic outcome might be "verbalizes a desire to stop taking drugs."

Example. For a newly diagnosed diabetic, the nurse may write this outcome: "correctly injects self with insulin prior to discharge." This goal may be unattainable for a variety of reasons—(1) the client may be discharged before the skill has been mastered, (2) the client may be unwilling or unable to achieve self-injection, or (3) the client may not require insulin therapy.

Determine Teaching Strategies. The teaching strategies utilized by the nurse should be individualized to the client's needs and the type of outcome desired. Knowledge outcomes frequently require the mastery of facts and concepts. These are most effectively taught by using written materials and audiovisual aids reinforced by discussion.

Skill outcomes are more likely to be achieved if the client is exposed to demonstration, discussion, practice, and reinforcement. Attitudes are more difficult to influence and to measure. However, discussion, role-modeling, and problem-solving experience assist the client in gaining insight into and accepting new attitudes.

The nurse may choose a variety of approaches, depending upon the client, the goal of teaching, the environment, available resources, time, and so on. The nurse may utilize individual or group instruction to accomplish learning outcomes.

Present Content. The nurse should identify the specific strategies and resources required to accomplish individual learning outcomes. Teaching methods previously described, when presented at the client's level of understanding, increase the possibility that new knowledge, skills, or attitudes will be acquired by the client. The pace of the program should be consistent with the client's ability to learn and should build on the client's previous knowledge. Learning is also facilitated when the teacher is a warm, accepting individual who encourages the active participation of the client. Retention is increased when (1) a number of the sense are involved in the learning process, (2) facts and skills are repeated, (3) the learner has the opportunity to apply the information, and (4) immediate feedback is provided.

Regardless of the strategy utilized in the teaching process, the interaction between the nurse and the client will affect the amount of learning that occurs. Supplemental teaching materials often enhance the client's ability to absorb content. Audiovisual aids, such as transparencies, films, filmstrips, slides, and audiotapes, may assist in the learning process. Models, posters, programmed instruction, and other printed materials may be utilized in specific instances. The nurse should be careful to review and assess these materials before using them. The materials selected should be appropriate, purposeful, and consistent with the goals of the teaching program. Additional resources should include sufficient time and personnel to assure that the client receives timely, pertinent information.

Evaluate Progress. The degree to which teaching has been effective may be measured by evaluating changes in the client's attitudes or skills. Attitudes are difficult to evaluate directly, since they are frequently subjective in nature. Therefore, changes in attitude are usually reflected in changes in behavior.

Example. Jane Adams, a 48 year old woman, had a colostomy performed five days ago. Initially, she refused to look at her stoma and cried when discussing the care involved. Following intensive teaching by the nurse and stomal therapist, Miss Adams was able to look at the stoma, and she asked questions about home care.

After teaching, the change in Miss Adams's attitude toward her colostomy was demonstrated by the changes in her behavior.

Learning may also be measured by comparison of the client's knowledge with the objectives of the teaching plan. If the outcome is "accurately measures and records radial pulse before taking Digoxin," the nurse may observe the client's technique while monitoring the pulse on the opposite side. The client's knowledge may be measured by verbal or written responses to questions designed to elicit the client's response.

Example. Using the teaching checklist in Figure 6–1, the nurse may evaluate the items under *Purpose* by asking the client:
1. Why is the TENS unit used?
2. What medications must be discontinued before surgery?
3. When should medication be requested?

The operation of the TENS unit may be evaluated by asking the client to demonstrate the mechanics of operating the unit.

Modify the Plan. After evaluating the teaching objectives, the nurse may decide either (1) to reteach the content or (2) to develop more realistic teaching objectives.

Utilization of Appropriate Resources

Appropriate resources are identified during the planning phase and are incorporated into the nursing order. The nurse must consider whether the nursing order is realistic for the client situation. The order should be practical in terms of equipment, financial factors, and human resources.

Equipment. It is necessary to be aware of the types of equipment readily available within an agency and in the community. The nurse should utilize the assistive device that is most useful, at the least cost, and yet acceptable to the client.

For example, a client with a potential impairment of skin integrity related to decreased mobility may be placed on a foam, air, or water mattress. Availability, cost, and acceptability will determine which device is selected.

Financial Factors. In addition to the selection of equipment, financial factors will influence the services available to the client. Clients with low income may be eligible for certain services, while other programs do not

HAMILTON HOSPITAL
Teaching Record
TENS

COMPLETE THE FOLLOWING:
Anticipated Surgical Procedure: _____

Obstacles to Learning:
☐ Vision   ☐ Language   ☐ None
☐ Hearing   ☐ Other _____

Contraindications for Use:
General   - ☐ Break in Skin   ☐ Pacemaker
              ☐ Skin Irritation   ☐ None

Medication - ☐ Valium   ☐ Morphine   ☐ None
              ☐ Steroids   ☐ Demerol

Following instruction, the patient/family will be able to:	INFORMATION PROVIDED DATE SIGNATURE	INFORMATION REINFORCED DATE SIGNATURE
PURPOSE:		
1. State reason for use of TENS		
2. Identify need to discontinue contraindicated medications before surgery.		
3. Initiate use of TENS unit before requesting medications.		
FUNCTION:		
1. Demonstrate mechanical operation (dial-mode switch)		
2. State function of		
intensity setting		
mode setting		
3. Describe placement and function of electrodes		
placement in OR		
duration		
source of power		
4. Verbalize need to modify setting for special circumstances:		
coughing		
change in activity		
5. Experience sensation of unit		

Figure 6–1 □ Post-op TENS teaching record. (Courtesy of Hamilton Hospital, Trenton, NJ.)
Illustration continued on following page

TEACHING RECORD - TENS   - 2 -

Following instruction, the patient/family will be able to:	INFORMATION PROVIDED DATE SIGNATURE	INFORMATION REINFORCED DATE SIGNATURE
SCOPE:		
1. Explain use of pain scale		
2. State options for trouble shooting unit.		
turn off		
notify nurse		
3. List method of managing:		
showers		
skin problems		
4. Explain discharge options:		
return to nurse		
rental home use		
return to hospital		

☐ Instruction sheet given - Signature _____

☐ Pain scale given -   Signature _____

COMMENTS:

_____
_____
_____
_____
_____
_____
_____
_____
_____

GS150
8/29/85

Figure 6–1 *Continued*

have income criteria. Social workers can often provide useful information about the financial aspects of available resources.

Human Resources. Human resources commonly utilized in the planning phase include health care personnel, family, and significant others. When formulating nursing orders, the nurse must evaluate the need for and availability of these human resources. The nurse must consider the family resources when making plans that might involve them. Aspects to consider include their commitment to assist in the situation, financial resources, and degree of understanding of the client's needs.

In summary, nursing orders should be realistic in the utilization of nursing staff, client, family, agency, and community resources.

Development of Nursing Orders

The nurse uses the scientific method in the development of nursing orders. This consists of (1) defining the problem (diagnosis), (2) identifying possible alternatives, and (3) selecting viable alternatives (nursing orders).

Once the nursing diagnoses and outcomes have been established, decisions are made on how to meet the outcomes and how to promote, maintain, or restore the client's health. The second step of the process is the generation of all possible solutions or alternatives. Successful nursing orders depend upon the nurse's ability to generate and choose alternatives that will most likely be effective. Both hypothesizing and brainstorming are useful in the identification of possible alternatives.

Hypothesizing

The nurse hypothesizes when predicting that certain alternatives are appropriate to reach the desired outcome. Nursing orders are proposed that (1) have been successful in the past in solving a particular problem and (2) are likely to be effective based on the client's knowledge, skills, or resources. This technique allows the nurse to apply scientific principles, develop creative approaches to problem-solving, and facilitate the delivery of individualized care.

Brainstorming

Brainstorming is a group technique utilized to generate ideas from more than one person. The purpose of this approach is to stimulate creative alternatives. An atmosphere of freedom and openness must be created for effective brainstorming to take place. Brainstorming can be done with the interdisciplinary team or among nursing staff. It may occur during a care planning session, team nursing meetings, or interdisciplinary team conferences. After all possible alternatives are developed, each should be judged in terms of its feasibility and probability of success. The nurse chooses those that are most appropriate for the client.

Whether approaches are developed by hypothesizing or brainstorming, they are translated into nursing orders and communicated both verbally and in the written plan of care.

Components of Nursing Orders

The nursing order provides the health care team with a blueprint for reaching the established outcomes and resolving the unhealthful response. A set of nursing orders should be written to accomplish each outcome. To be effective, the nursing orders must be written as clearly and concisely as possible. To avoid confusion or repetition of activities, they should describe who will implement them. When nursing orders are dependent on previous orders, they should be numbered to designate sequence. All orders should consist of

- □ Date
- □ Precise action verb and modifiers
- □ Specifications of "who, what, where, when, how, and how much"
- □ Modifications in standard therapy
- □ Signature

Date

All nursing orders should be dated to identify the date of origin.

Action Verbs and Modifiers

All nursing orders should clearly communicate the expected activities. Employing action verbs is useful in defining the specific actions. Verbs that are not precise create confusion for the caregiver. For example, if the order is "teach colostomy care," the nurse could (1) demonstrate the steps used in applying a colostomy pouch; (2) identify the equipment required in colostomy care; (3) provide printed instructions and discuss their content with the client; or (4) ask the client to perform a return demonstration. In this example, the verb "teach" is not precise. A more specific verb gives clear directions to the nurse.

Who, What, Where, When, How, and How Much

Specifications of "who, what, where, when, how, and how much" are necessary to make the nursing order meaningful. In the example "irrigate wound vigorously," the implementor needs to know

□ Which wound—perhaps the client has more than one.
□ Who will irrigate—the nurse, client, or family?
□ When to irrigate—prior to physical therapy? Once a day? Each time the dressing is changed?
□ How to irrigate—vigorously by pouring the solution? Using a bulb syringe? With normal saline, peroxide, Betadine (povidone-iodine), or antibiotic solution?

Putting all of this together, the nursing orders may read
"4/29—Irrigate lower abdominal incision at 10 A.M., 6 P.M., and 2 A.M.
Using a bulb syringe, irrigate vigorously with neomycin solution, followed by normal saline.
Demonstrate wound irrigation technique to client and family members.
Replace with a dressing using two gauze sponges and one 8 in × 8 in pad.
Use paper tape (client's skin is very sensitive.)"
The nurse should also include the duration of time, when indicated. For example, "OOB in chair for 30 minutes tid."

Modifications in Treatment

If routine procedures are spelled out in procedure manuals or protocols, the title of the procedure may be used in the nursing orders to eliminate writing the entire procedure. Some examples of this might be "tracheostomy care" or "urinary catheter care." If modifications of the procedure need to be made, they are to be included in the nursing order. Using the example of "tracheostomy care," the nursing order may read
"Tracheostomy care at least once a shift and when there is a noticeable build-up of secretions.
Do not change trach strings. To be changed by MD only."
A modification of Hickman catheter care might read

"Perform Hickman catheter care three times weekly—Monday, Wednesday, and Friday.

Do not use Betadine—client is allergic."

Signature

The final component of the nursing order is a signature. It reflects the nurse's personal and legal accountability. The signature allows coworkers (1) to give feedback on the effectiveness of the order, (2) to obtain clarification, and (3) to explore the rationale for the order (Carnevali, 1983).

STAGE IV—DOCUMENTATION: THE NURSING CARE PLAN

The fourth and final stage of the planning phase is recording the nursing diagnoses, outcomes, and nursing orders in an organized fashion. This is accomplished through documentation on the nursing care plan.

Definition

The nursing care plan is an information processing, receiving, sending, and evaluating center initiated by the professional nurse (Ryan, 1973). The format of the care plan assists the nurse to process the information gathered during the assessment and diagnostic phases. The care plan acts as a receiving center when the nurse uses it to document the results of the planning phase. It facilitates communication by the sending of pertinent information. It also provides a mechanism for the evaluation of care provided. Development of pertinent care plans requires the nurse to have assessment, diagnostic, communication, and judgment skills.

Purposes

Nursing care plans are written in a variety of settings and are designed to promote quality care by facilitating (1) individualized care, (2) continuity of care, (3) communication, and (4) evaluation (Bower, 1982).

Text continued on page 163

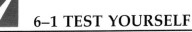

6–1 TEST YOURSELF

IDENTIFICATION OF CORRECTLY AND INCORRECTLY WRITTEN ORDERS

The following is a list of orders. Decide whether each order is written correctly or incorrectly. If written incorrectly, identify the reason.

	Correct	**Incorrect**	**Reason**

1. Make the client comfortable

2. OOB in chair for ½ hour bid

3. Teach about diabetes management

4. No evidence of signs of infection

5. Force fluids

6. Teach client to do ten ankle pumps q1h while awake

7. Hickman catheter care daily

6–1 TEST YOURSELF □ ANSWERS

	Correct	Incorrect	Reason
1. Make the client comfortable		✔	It is not clear what the nurse is supposed to do to make the client comfortable
2. OOB in chair for ½ hour bid	✔		
3. Teach about diabetes management		✔	Imprecise
4. No evidence of signs of infection		✔	This is an outcome
5. Force fluids		✔	Does not specify amount per shift
6. Teach client to do ten ankle pumps q1h while awake	✔		
7. Hickman catheter care daily	✔		

6–2 TEST YOURSELF

DEVELOPMENT OF NURSING ORDERS

Helen O'Brien is a 47 year old white female admitted to your unit. Your assessment reveals the following vital signs: T = 101°F, B/P = 96/70 mm Hg, P = 110 beats/minute, R = 18 breaths/minute (no abnormal breath sounds), height = 5 ft, 5 in, weight = 96 lb. Helen's skin is dry and pale with decreased turgor, and she has an emaciated appearance. She has no obvious decubiti; however, you note reddened areas on her coccyx and elbows.

She has full range of motion but is unable to walk without assistance, since she is often weak and dizzy. Helen indicates that she has fallen twice at home; however, there is no evidence of injury. She is alert and oriented but is obviously tense throughout the interview. She moves her hands continuously and changes position frequently. She cries intermittently and is particularly tearful when her husband is mentioned. She states "I'm not surprised this happened—I knew I'd get sick if I didn't eat more." She indicates that she has been unable to eat or sleep since the death of her husband two months ago. Helen shares that she is extremely lonely and feels worried and helpless most of the time.

Lab data reveal
    CBC: decreased Hgb and RBC, increased hematocrit
    Urinalysis: concentrated dark amber urine with increased specific gravity; urine culture negative
    Chest x-ray and EKG: normal

Develop nursing orders for each nursing diagnosis and its outcomes.

Nursing Diagnoses	Outcomes	Nursing Orders
Alteration in nutrition (less than body requirements) related to decreased caloric intake	Consumes 2000 calories daily	
Ineffective individual coping related to feelings of loneliness and helplessness	By the time of discharge, identifies available support systems	
Potential for injury related to dizziness and weakness	Calls for assistance before ambulating; throughout hospitalization, no evidence of injury	
Sleep pattern disturbance related to insomnia secondary to grieving	Sleeps four hours each night without interruption	
Potential impairment of skin integrity related to decreased nutrition and hydration	Throughout hospitalization, no evidence of skin breakdown; drinks 2500 ml daily	

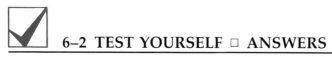

Nursing Diagnoses	Outcome	Nursing Orders
Alteration in nutrition (less than body requirements) related to decreased caloric intake	Consumes 2000 calories daily	1. Determine food likes and dislikes 2. Offer small frequent feedings every four hours at 8 A.M., 12 P.M., 4 P.M., and 8 P.M. 3. Encourage the client to drink milkshakes at 10 A.M. and 6 P.M. 4. Closely observe the client's food and fluid intake 5. Give the client positive feedback for adhering to prescribed diet
Ineffective individual coping related to feelings of loneliness and helplessness	By the time of discharge, identifies available support systems	1. Encourage the client to verbalize her feelings 2. Let her know you will listen and accept what she is expressing 3. Allow her to cry if desired; stay with and support her or provide privacy for brief periods 4. Assist the client to identify available support systems in the community 5. Support the client when she is making choices
Potential for injury related to dizziness and weakness	Calls for assistance before ambulating Throughout hospitalization, no evidence of injury	1. Encourage use of railings when in bathroom and hall 2. Keep room free of obstacles 3. Side rails up at all times 4. Keep items within reach on bedside stand (telephone, call bell) 5. Ask client to call for help before getting OOB
Sleep pattern disturbance related to insomnia secondary to grieving	Sleeps four hours each night without interruption	If client cannot sleep: 1. Provide a quiet peaceful time for resting 2. Provide a nighttime routine to encourage sleep 3. Interact with client for short periods during night hours 4. Reduce caffeine intake during the evening hours 5. Discourage sleeping during the day
Potential impairment of skin integrity related to decreased nutrition and hydration	Throughout hospitalization, no evidence of skin breakdown Drinks 2500 ml daily	1. Inspect the skin for reddened areas q shift 2. Place egg-crate mattress on bed 3. Massage bony prominences gently with lotion q4h

The care plan serves as a blueprint for directing nursing activities toward the fulfillment of the client's health needs. It provides a mechanism for the provision of consistent, coordinated care. The care plan is utilized as a communication tool among nurses and other members of the health care team. In addition, it guides the nurse in the evaluation of the effectiveness of care delivered.

Characteristics

Regardless of the setting in which they are written, nursing care plans have certain desirable characteristics. They are
  1. Written by a registered nurse
  2. Initialed following the first contact with the client
  3. Readily available
  4. Current

Written by a Registered Nurse

The American Nurses' Association, Joint Commission, and many nurse practice acts have addressed the development of nursing care plans. They have defined the role of the registered nurse as including responsibility for the initiation of the care plan. Based on educational preparation, the registered nurse is the most qualified person to complete this function. The client and other health care providers should be involved in the development of the plan. The client may contribute by defining and validating outcomes and nursing orders.

Example. Frankie Cattner, a six year old boy, has been seen in the school nurse's office twice within the last month. Each visit was precipitated by an acute asthmatic attack. After questioning Frankie, the school nurse determines that each of the attacks occurred shortly after he spent the day with a friend who has six cats. Frankie and the nurse agree to a mutual goal of the reduction or elimination of these attacks. They also agree to the following approach: Frankie will invite his friend to play at his house or in public parks.

The involvement of the client in this situation enhances the probability of successful resolution of his problem.

The nurse may also utilize the assistance of other health care providers in the development of the nursing care plan. These may include LPNs, aides, and members of other disciplines, such as social services or speech therapy.

Example. Glenn Weiser, a 57 year old man, is being followed at home by the visiting nurse. He is aphasic as a result of a stroke. His sister manages his daily care and verbalizes her frustration over Glenn's inability to communicate his needs. The nurse presents the problem to a speech therapist, who recommends the use of a picture board. This enables the client to point to the things he needs and decreases his frustration.

In addition to participating in the development of the plan, other health care providers may be utilized in its implementation. Specific nursing activities may be delegated to other nursing personnel, such as LPNs or nursing assistants. However, the responsibility and accountability for the initiation of the care plan rest with the registered nurse.

Initiation Following First Contact

The nursing care plan is most effective when it is initiated after the nurse's first contact with the client. Immediately after obtaining the data base, the nurse should begin to document actual or potential diagnoses, outcomes, and orders. A partially developed plan will assist the nurse to focus on the client's needs. Additional interaction with the client may result in further development and refinement of the plan of care.

The nurse who obtains the data base has the most information about the client. Therefore, it is more likely that this nurse will be able to develop a comprehensive plan. Occasionally a comprehensive data base may not be collected because of time constraints, condition of the client, or the initiation of treatment modalities. In this situation the nurse may

1. Develop a preliminary plan based on the available information
2. Gather the absent data during subsequent contacts with the client
3. Refine the preliminary plan
4. Delegate the responsibility for obtaining the absent data and refining the preliminary plan to another registered nurse

The trend toward decreasing the length of stay for hospitalized clients emphasizes the importance of initiating the care plan on the first contact with the client. By identifying the client's needs at the time of admission, the nurse promotes efficient and coordinated care.

Readily Available

The nursing care plan should be readily available to all personnel involved in the care of the client. It may be located on the client's medical record, at the bedside, or in a centralized location. Ready access to the care plan facilitates its usefulness and its value as a communication tool.

Current

Since the nursing care plan is the blueprint for directing the client's care, it must contain current information. Therefore, it is essential that all components of the nursing care plan be updated frequently. Nursing diagnoses, outcomes, and orders that are no longer valid are either eliminated or revised. The method of updating the care plan varies with the type of nursing care plan format utilized and agency policy.

The continuity and individualization of the care plan may be jeopardized when it is not current.

Example. Elaine Conner is a hospitalized client whose IV infusion infiltrated three days ago. The nurse made a diagnosis of "alteration in comfort: pain related to edema in right forearm." The nursing orders include "warm soaks via K pad for ½ hour, tid at 10 A.M., 4 P.M., and 10 P.M." Today when a different nurse attempts to apply the soaks as ordered. Elaine informs her that they were discontinued yesterday.

As a result of an outdated care plan, the nurse's time was not utilized effectively. Furthermore, the client may lose confidence in the nurse's ability to deliver appropriate care.

Components

The nursing care plan may be structured in several ways, depending on the system in use in the agency. However, the components of the nursing care plan usually consist of
1. Nursing diagnoses
2. Outcomes
3. Nursing orders
Each of these components has been previously described in detail.

The nursing care plan is frequently supplemented by the use of a Kardex. This form usually consists of a checklist of frequently ordered medical and nursing functions (Figure 6–2). Diagnostic studies and treatments may be recorded on the Kardex in specific areas. The nursing implications associated with these modalities are defined in the nursing care plan.

Example. The doctor orders a myelogram utilizing Amipaque (metriza-
mide). The nurse places the order on the Kardex, assesses the client's
knowledge of the procedure, and develops the care plan as follows.

Nursing Diagnosis	Outcome	Orders
Knowledge deficit related to scheduled diagnostic study	Explains the usual pre- and postmyelogram care No evidence of headache postmyelogram	1. Review booklet on myelograms with client on evening of 6/11 2. Explain pre- and post-myelogram guidelines for fluid intake and position 3. Encourage client to verbalize feelings about the outcome of the myelogram

Types of Care Plans

There are several different types of care plans in use. Those that are most
common include individualized, standardized, modified standardized,
and computerized care plans.

Figure 6–2 □ Kardex documentation form. (Courtesy of Mercer Medical Center, Trenton,
NJ.)

Individualized

Individualized care plans are forms divided into columns with the usual headings of nursing diagnoses, client goals or outcomes, and nursing orders.

Advantages. The individualized care plan enables the documentation of the nursing diagnoses, outcomes, and orders that are most pertinent to a particular client. No extraneous or inapplicable information is included in the care plan.

Disadvantages. The individualized care plan is time-consuming to develop. This will be explored later in the chapter.

Standardized

Standardized care plans have been introduced into several types of agencies to facilitate the preparation and use of care plans. According to Mayers (1983), "a standard care plan is a specific protocol of care that is appropriate for patients who are experiencing the usual or predictable problems associated with a given diagnosis or disease process." Standardized care plans consists of actual, potential, or possible nursing diagnoses, outcomes, and interventions that are printed in a care plan format. The care plans may be developed by the nursing staff of a particular agency or may be derived from the literature. Sources of published standardized care plans include journal articles or books. Table 6–1 is an example of a standardized care plan.

Standardized care plans may be used in one of two ways: (1) they may be placed in a centrally located area and referred to by nurses when developing individualized care plans, or (2) they may be placed directly on the Kardex, dated, and signed.

Advantages. The advantages of standardized care plans include the following.

1. They are usually developed by clinical experts who have carefully researched the literature. Therefore, the standardized care plans become the standards of care for clients with a given diagnosis. In the process, they are educating nurses who are not familiar with a certain medical or nursing diagnosis.

2. They reduce the amount of time spent in writing nursing care plans. This increases the efficiency of nursing care planning.

Disadvantages. The major disadvantage of standardized care plans is that they do not provide for the individual differences in clients with similar

TABLE 6–1 □ **STANDARDIZED CARE PLAN—
NORMAL POSTPARTUM VAGINAL DELIVERY**

Nursing Diagnosis	Outcomes	Nursing Plan
1. Potential fluid volume deficit related to postpartum hemorrhage	BP normal for client No evidence of hemorrhage by the time of discharge	1. Assess lochia for amount 2. Assess fundus q shift 3. Teach client how to perform fundal exam and characteristics of normal lochia
2. Potential for injury related to infection	Temp within normal limits No evidence of infection during hospitalization	1. Assess lochia for odor 2. Teach client pericare 3. Check temp qid and as needed

3. Potential alteration in comfort: pain related to edema secondary to episiotomy, uterine cramps, breast engorgement	Expresses comfort within one hour after initiation of comfort measures
	Initiates comfort measures for breast engorgement
		1. Assess location, intensity, and duration of pain
		2. Administer analgesics as ordered prn
		3. Apply ice to incision prn
		4. Sitz bath prn
		5. Teach comfort-promoting exercises
		6. For bottle feeding:
		  (a) Administer suppressants as ordered
		  (b) Instruct in application of well-fitting bra or binder
		  (c) Apply ice packs to breasts for 15 minutes q 1–3 hours

4. Potential alteration in urine elimination related to pain, decreased fluid intake, or bladder distention	Voids 180–200 ml at one time within 6–12 hours postdelivery	In addition to comfort measure listed above:
		1. Measure output for three voidings
		2. Encourage fluid intake to 2500 ml daily
		  7–3 1500 ml
		  3–11 500 ml
		  11–7 500 ml
		3. Catheterize per Dr.'s orders
		4. Check for bladder distention q4h until client has voided
		5. Teach to report signs and symptoms of distention

5. Potential alteration in bowel elimination related to pain, fear of pain, decreased mobility, and decreased oral intake	Bowel movement by third postpartum day	In addition to comfort measures listed above: 1. Administer stool softeners or laxatives as ordered 2. Fleets enema by third day if needed 3. Instruct in planning high fiber diet with fresh fruits

TABLE 6–1 □ **STANDARDIZED CARE PLAN—
NORMAL POSTPARTUM VAGINAL DELIVERY** *Continued*

Nursing Diagnosis	Outcomes	Nursing Plan
6. Knowledge deficit related to newborn care	Demonstrates knowledge of newborn care prior to discharge (diaper change, bath, feeding technique, and taking temp)	1. Assess level of knowledge 2. Show nursery films and encourage discussion—date done: 3. Instruct in newborn care and assess mother's knowledge —date done: 4. Arrange return demonstration of newborn care—date done:
7. Potential alteration in parenting related to lack of parental-infant attachment	Demonstrates beginning parental-infant attachment prior to discharge by eye contact, touching, and positive verbalizations about the baby	1. Encourage spouse or significant other to become involved in newborn care 2. Point out baby's positive characteristics and behaviors 3. Act as role model to demonstrate positive interactions with infant 4. Encourage mother to keep infant with her 5. In absence of bonding refer to social service for discharge follow-up 6. Attend parenting class

problems. For example, the first part of the nursing diagnosis may be appropriate, but the etiology may not apply. Predetermined outcomes do not reflect the client's input. The nursing orders may contain interventions that do not relate to an individual client.

Modified Standardized

Modified standardized care plans allow for individualization. The nursing diagnoses, outcomes, or interventions may be individualized through the use of blank spaces. See Table 6–2 for an example of a modified standardized care plan. Additional standardized and modified standardized care plans are found in Appendix F.

In addition to modification of the standardized care plan, the nurse may cross off items that do not apply to the client or add additional nursing diagnoses, outcomes, and orders.

Advantages. Modified standardized care plans offer the advantages of both individualized and standardized care plans. They provide informa-

TABLE 6–2 □ **MODIFIED STANDARDIZED CARE PLAN—
TOTAL HIP REPLACEMENT (POST-OP)**

Nursing Diagnosis	Outcomes	Nursing Plan
1. Potential for injury related to □ Risk of dislocation	At time of discharge, demonstrates healing with extremity in proper alignment	1. Keep ____ hip abducted at all times (specify) (with two pillows between legs). 2. Keep hips flexed at all times (no greater than 45° until ordered). 3. Elevate ____ leg on pillow. 4. Foot of bed gatched. 5. Keep HOB (head of bed) elevated 15–45° at all times. 6. Neurovascular checks of *both* extremities q ____ h × ____ h, then q ____ h. 7. Gentle foot-ankle exercises qlh. *Start first post-op day.* 8. OOB/chair (specify). No weight bearing ____ leg. Place 1–2 pillows on the wheelchair to elevate hips. Never place the legs of the wheelchair level with the seat of the chair. 9. When changing bed linens, HOB and legs flat, two pillows between legs, logroll onto operated side. 10. Bilateral ace bandages × 48 hr—remove q shift, inspect extremity, and reapply. 11. TED stocking third post-op day; knee-high on operated leg, thigh-high on unoperated leg. 12. OOB → bathroom—use elevated toilet seat or elevated commode. Elevate HOB 20° before putting on bedpan. Fracture pan prn.
□ Decreased mobility	No loss of muscle tone/strength in unaffected extremities	1. Initiate ROM exercises for unaffected extremities. 2. Quad sets and gluteal sets according to post-op protocol.
□ Infectious process	Throughout hospitalization, no S & S of infection in incision	1. Observe dressing. 2. Report drainage.

TABLE 6–2 □ **MODIFIED STANDARDIZED CARE PLAN—
TOTAL HIP REPLACEMENT (POST-OP)** *Continued*

Nursing Diagnosis	Outcomes	Nursing Plan
2. Alteration in comfort: pain related to inflammatory process/edema	No evidence of unusual edema at time of discharge	1. Monitor extremity q _____ h × _____ h for unusual edema. 2. Evaluate extremity for constriction by ace bandage/TED stocking. 3. Neurovascular checks q _____ h × _____ h. 4. Maintain suction drainage system (specify). 5. Chart amount and consistency of drainage q shift. 6. Change dressing daily and prn (as ordered by MD).
3. Potential impairment of skin integrity related to decreased mobility	No evidence of skin breakdown at time of discharge	1. Initial turning schedule: turn q _____ h (specify). 2. Massage bony prominences q _____ h. 3. Keep skin clean and dry at all times. 4. Monitor nutritional and fluid intake. 5. Relieve pressure on both heels with bilateral heel protectors.
4. Potential alteration in health maintenance related to lack of knowledge re: postdischarge care	Prior to discharge: Demonstrates proper positioning and transfer techniques Verbalizes discharge instructions regarding activity	1. Have patient demonstrate transfer techniques. 2. Reinforce information given by MD, physical therapy. 3. Stress that the patient *should not* (a) Flex hip more than 90° (b) Sit on low chair, stool, or toilet seat (c) Bend to tie shoes (d) Cross legs when sitting, standing, or lying (e) Get up from a chair without moving to the edge first (f) Lie on "good side" without a pillow between legs (g) Pick up any objects from the floor or reach into lower cupboard or drawers.

tion specific to a particular client and require less time to complete. Additionally, since they outline the accepted standards of care, they enhance the quality of the delivery and documentation of care. A study by Nodhturft and MacMullen (1982) found that modified standardized care plans "became an effective tool for the delivery of high levels of nursing care and the documentation of nursing care delivered."

Disadvantages. If not correctly used, modified standardized care plans can have some of the same disadvantages as standardized plans. Although blank spaces are provided, the user may not utilize them. Therefore the plan does not reflect the client's individual needs. In addition, the modified plan may contain extraneous information that does not reflect the client's needs.

Computerized

The basic elements of care plan systems, nursing diagnoses, outcomes, and nursing orders are also present in automatic systems. The nursing care plan may be prepared at a terminal in the client's room or in a central location. Once data are validated and entered, a printed version may be generated daily, each shift, or on demand (Figure 6–3). There are a number of mechanisms by which care plans are generated. Three commonly used systems are (1) standardized plans based on the medical diagnosis, (2) standardized plans based on the nursing diagnosis, and (3) individually constructed plans.

Medical Diagnoses. In these systems, the computer provides the nurse with nursing diagnoses, outcomes, and nursing orders commonly associated with the medical diagnoses. These are very similar to the printed standardized care plans discussed earlier. The nurse who is formulating the plan selects the appropriate items from the standardized data base. Additional diagnoses, outcomes, and orders may be entered to reflect other concerns of the client.

Nursing Diagnoses. Other computerized systems are more directly associated with the specific nursing diagnoses identified at the time of the detailed nursing assessment. The computer lists each problem, and the nurse defines outcomes and nursing orders by selecting from a menu of appropriate choices. The nurse may add other specific outcomes and orders for an individual client, if appropriate. Some systems are constructed to allow clients to participate actively in the selection of outcomes and appropriate interventions. The nurse assists clients to choose outcomes or orders that they feel will best meet their needs. Selections are

```
                         P A T I E N T   C A R E   P L A N
        GENERAL HOSPITAL          5/16/84  11:41AM              PAGE    1

                              │TRN-09        000187023 2555555      TRN
                              │TESTPAT JACK                    SEX: M
                              │ADM: 5/15/84       SRV:URO  SMK: N
                              │DOB: 10/06/21 62 COND: G  LEVEL: 1
                              │HT: 5/11  F/I        WT: 180/000 P/O
                              │10000 INTERNIST OTHER
                              │ALG: PENICILLIN
                              │DX: NEPHROLITHIASIS
```

KNOWLEDGE DEFICIT RELATED
TO SURGICAL EXPERIENCE

```
        OUTCOME:          Describes type of surgery
        OUTCOME:          States usual pre-op preparation
        OUTCOME:          Identifies usual post-op routine
        OUTCOME:          Verbalizes feelings about impending surgery

        INTERVENTION:     Assess knowledge of surgery and explore past
                          surgical experience(s) at the time of admission

        INTERVENTION:     Review surgical routine (preps, meds, dressing)

        INTERVENTION:     Reinforce pre-operative teaching
                          re: Sequence of events on day of surgery (pre-op
                              stretcher to O.R., R.R. return to room/ICU)
                              Post-op equipment (dsg., I.V., tubes)
                              Provisions for relief of pain and other
                              symptoms (include need to request and frequency
                              limitations)
                              Turning, coughing and deep breathing
                              Incentive spirometry if ordered
                              Change in bowel/bladder functions
                              Progressive diet changes
                              Progressive self care
```

Figure 6–3 □ Computerized care plan. (Courtesy of HBO & Company, Atlanta, GA. All rights reserved.)

made from a menu that includes appropriate outcomes or nursing orders (Wesseling, 1980).

Individually Constructed. In these systems, the nurse develops the care plan in a fashion similar to that used in a manual individualized plan. The nurse is not prompted to focus on specific diagnoses but uses a menu to select those diagnoses, outcomes, and orders that apply to the individual client. Additional outcomes or interventions not identified in the menu may also be added when necessary.

Most computerized care planning systems facilitate frequent updating of the plan. The nurse identifies problems that have been resolved, and they are eliminated from the plan. Other options may include (1) revision of diagnoses, outcomes, and orders to reflect the changing status of the client or (2) addition of new diagnoses, outcomes, and orders. Printed care plans, which are a permanent part of the medical record, document the client's progress as reflected by the changing plan of care.

Computerized care plans increase the potential for accurate and thorough documentation of the delivery of care. The computer identifies specific nursing approaches listed on the plan and prompts the nurse to document the outcome of the intervention. This process also encourages frequent review of the plan as well as modification, when appropriate.

SUMMARY

The development of nursing orders is the third stage of the planning phase of the nursing process. Nursing orders define the activities that assist the client to achieve desired outcomes. Nursing orders are consistent with the plan of care, based on scientific principles, and individualized to the specific client situation. They are also used to provide a safe and therapeutic environment. Additionally, nursing orders include teaching-learning opportunities for the client and the utilization of appropriate resources.

Nursing orders are developed through a scientific approach and include date, precise action verbs, specific aspects of interventions, and modifications in standard therapy. The registered nurse is responsible and accountable for the development of nursing orders.

The fourth stage of the planning phase consists of documentation of the plan on a nursing care plan. Care plans may be individualized, standardized, or computerized. Much time is wasted when care plans are not developed. Nurses who are unfamiliar with the client's care may spend time in reviewing the client's record and asking questions of other nursing personnel or of the client. This hit or miss approach leads to a great deal of wasted effort and inefficient care, which could be avoided by documentation of the plan. Care plans are necessary to provide a framework for the delivery of care and to ensure continuity.

References

American Nurses' Association: Standards of Nursing Practice. St. Louis: American Nurses' Association, 1973.
Bower F: The Process of Planning Nursing Care. 3rd ed. St. Louis: CV Mosby, 1982.
Carnevali D: Nursing Care Planning: Diagnosis and Management. 3rd ed. Philadelphia: JB Lippincott, 1983.
Mayers M: A Systematic Approach to the Nursing Care Plan. 3rd ed. Norwalk, Conn: Appleton-Century-Crofts, 1983.
Nodhturft V and MacMullen J: Standardized nursing care plans. Nursing Management 33–42, October 1982.
Ryan B: Nursing care plans: a systems approach to developing criteria for planning and evaluation. Journal of Nursing Administration. 50–58, May–June 1973.
Wesseling E: Automating the nursing history and care plan. In Zielstorff R: Computers in Nursing. Rockville, Md: Aspen, 1980.

Bibliography

Blount M and Sanborn C: Standard plan for care and discharge. American Journal of Nursing 1394–1396, November 1984.

Fraher J: Nursing diagnoses and care plans in critical care. Critical Care Nurse November/December, 1983.

Hanson R: The nursing history and care plan: a throw-away? In Marriner A: Nursing Process. St. Louis: CV Mosby, 1979.

Hinson I, Nettie S, and Clapp P: An automated Kardex and care plan. Nursing Management Vol 15, No 7, July 1984.

Little D and Carnevali D: Nursing care plans: let's be practical about them. In Marriner A: Nursing Process. St. Louis: CV Mosby, 1979.

Marriner A: The Nursing Process: A Scientific Approach to Nursing Care. 3rd ed. St. Louis: CV Mosby, 1983.

McConnell E: How nursing care plans help you. Nursing Life January/February, Vol 2, 1982.

Stevens B: Why won't nurses write nursing care plans? In Marriner A. Nursing Process. St. Louis: CV Mosby, 1979.

7

Implementation

Implementation is the initiation of the nursing care plan to achieve specific outcomes. The implementation phase begins after the care plan has been developed and focuses on the initiation of those nursing orders that assist the client to accomplish desired outcomes. Specific nursing interventions are implemented to modify the factors contributing to the client's problem.

Nurses implement plans of care in a variety of settings. A survey conducted by the American Nurses' Association in 1977 identified the percentage of registered nurses practicing in different settings (Kelly, 1981). The results were as follows:

Hospital	61.4%
Nursing home	8.1%
Public health	7.9%
Physician's office	7.1%
Student health	4.2%
Nursing education	3.9%
Private duty	2.9%
Occupational health	2.5%
Self-employed	0.5%
Placement service	0.4%
Other	1.0%

The survey also indicated the percentage of registered nurses employed by type of position. These are indicated below:

General duty/staff	63.6%

Head nurse	8.7%
Supervisor	6.8%
Instructor	4.9%
Administrator	4.9%
Consultant	0.5%
Other	10.5%
Not reported	0.1%

These figures demonstrate that the largest number of registered nurses remain employed in hospitals as staff nurses. Projections for the future predict that hospitalized clients will be sicker and that their length of stay will be shorter. These two factors are the result of

□ Advanced medical knowledge, which allows the management of complex medical problems;
□ Technological advances resulting in sophisticated treatment modalities;
□ Increased regulation of inpatient facilities requiring that clients meet particular criteria prior to admission;
□ Changes in reimbursement systems such as Diagnostic Related Groupings (DRGs), which place a premium on timely treatment and discharge;
□ Utilization review activities, which monitor the client's length of stay and encourage discharge at the earliest opportunity.

DRGs and the utilization review process result in the discharge of clients into the community earlier than traditionally seen. The level of care required in the home or in ambulatory care settings is increasing. These trends are resulting in a decline in the hospital census and an increased demand for nurses in community health settings.

Regardless of the settings in which nurses practice, the nursing process is utilized to provide care to clients. The nurse utilizes three stages to complete the implementation phase. These are (1) preparation, (2) intervention, and (3) documentation.

STAGE 1—PREPARATION

The first stage of the implementation phase requires the nurse to prepare for the initiation of nursing actions. This preparation involves a series of activities, including the following:

1. Reviewing the nursing actions identified in the planning phase
2. Analyzing the nursing knowledge and skills required.
3. Recognizing the potential complications associated with specific nursing activities
4. Determining and providing necessary resources

5. Preparing an environment conducive to the types of activities required

6. Identifying and considering the legal and ethical concerns associated with potential nursing interventions

Reviewing Anticipated Nursing Actions

Nursing orders are designed to promote, maintain, or restore the client's health. When preparing to implement a nursing order, the nurse should review it to ensure that it remains current and includes certain desirable characteristics. These were identified in Chapter 6 and are summarized below:

Nursing actions should

☐ Be consistent with the plan of care
☐ Be based on scientific principles
☐ Be individualized to the specific situation
☐ Be used to provide a safe and therapeutic environment
☐ Employ teaching-learning opportunities for the client
☐ Include utilization of appropriate resources

Nursing actions that include these characteristics help to ensure that the client will receive quality nursing care.

Analyzing Knowledge and Skills Required

After reviewing the orders in the plan of care, the nurse should identify the level of knowledge and types of skills required for implementation. This allows the nurse to determine the person who is best qualified to perform the required activities. It may be a member of the nursing department—clinical nurse specialist, registered nurse, licensed practical nurse, or nursing assistant.

Example. Missy Stevens is a 16 year old with a fractured femur. Her pre-op nursing orders include "teach coughing and deep breathing 5/8 P.M."

The nurse recognizes that this order requires knowledge of the relationship between adequate ventilation and effective removal of secretions and postoperative respiratory complications. The order also requires skills to explain the rationale, demonstrate the procedure, and encourage the client to practice coughing and deep breathing preoperatively. The nurse determines that the practical nurse who is caring for Missy is capable of initiating this order.

Personnel from other disciplines may also be involved in the implementation of nursing orders. They may include the respiratory therapist, dietician, social worker, or speech therapist.

Example. Zack Cronin is an elderly client recently transferred to an extended care facility after a total hip replacement. He often verbalizes frustration over his inability to put his own shoes and socks on. Nursing orders for Mr. Cronin include "teach client to put on socks and shoes using long-handled shoe horn."

The nurse recognizes that this order requires specific knowledge about total hip surgery, body mechanics, and the use of assistive devices. In this case, an occupational therapist will be requested to assist in teaching Mr. Cronin.

Recognizing Potential Complications

The initiation of certain nursing procedures may involve potential risks to the client. The nurse needs to be aware of the most common complications associated with the activities specified in the client's nursing orders. This allows the nurse to initiate preventive approaches that decrease the risk to the client.

Example. Pat Ponticiello is a 35 year old woman who is three days post-op following an abdominal hysterectomy. Her catheter has been removed and nursing orders include "ambulate to bathroom twice each shift; utilize nursing measures to encourage voiding—e.g., running water; check for bladder distention q4h (10 A.M., 2 P.M., 6 P.M., etc.); catheterize q8h prn."

In this case, both bladder distention and catheterization pose a risk for the client. Distention may result in an atonic bladder, while infection may be associated with catheter insertion. Based on this knowledge, the nurse palpates and percusses the abdomen carefully to identify the presence of distention. Should catheterization be necessary, the nurse utilizes meticulous sterile technique to avoid the introduction of organisms at the time of insertion.

Other less invasive procedures may also result in complications for the client.

Example. Sarah Johnson is a 56 year old woman with a medical diagnosis of cancer of the liver. One of Sarah's nursing diagnoses is "alteration in nutrition less than body requirements related to anorexia secondary to chemotherapy." The physician orders 2500 ml of tube feedings daily Associated nursing orders include "monitor continuous tube feedings q2h (even hours); check tube placement q shift—8 A.M., 4 P.M., 12 mn, and prn."

In this case, the nurse is aware of the potential for aspiration in the client with a feeding tube. Based on this knowledge, the position of the tube is monitored to prevent or detect dislodgement and associated aspiration of feedings. The nurse also utilizes other techniques to avoid diarrhea. These include dilution of feedings to half-strength, use of continuous rather than intermittent feedings, and maintenance of constant flow rate with the assistance of a feeding pump.

The client may also be at risk as a result of the nurse's failure to prevent common complications associated with the client's illness or treatment modalities. For example, this is typified by the pulmonary and embolic complications that may occur following surgery. Nursing orders designed to prevent these problems include

"Encourage coughing and deep breathing q2h (even hours)."
"Turn and reposition q2h (even hours)."
"Apply antiembolism stockings."
"Remind client to do at least ten ankle pumps per hour."

A common hazard in the elderly client is altered skin integrity resulting from prolonged immobility. The nurse frequently initiates orders to minimize the risk to these clients. They may include

"Apply egg-crate (foam) mattress to bed."
"Turn q2h (odd hours) as specified on turning schedule."
"Massage bony prominences with lotion after turning."
"Bathe qod (even dates)—add Alpha Keri to water."
"Apply transparent dressing to reddened area on sacrum—change q4 days and prn."

The preventive approaches outlined above reflect a comprehensive nursing effort to protect the client in these circumstances. These may be necessary until the client is completely recovered, immobility is decreased, or the client is able to initiate such measures independently.

Providing Necessary Resources

When preparing to initiate nursing actions, a number of concerns about resources should be addressed. These include time, personnel, and equipment.

Time

There are a variety of time considerations that affect the nurse's ability to implement the plan. First, the nurse must be careful to select the appropriate time for the initiation of specific interventions.

Example. Donna Kelsey is an 18 year old recovering from abdominal surgery, which was performed two days ago, for a perforated appendix. Nursing orders include "teach client to do dressing change on 1/3." The nurse enters Donna's room to begin teaching and finds her walking around the room, clutching her abdomen. Donna indicates that she has "gas pains."

In this case, the nurse recognizes that this is not the appropriate time to begin teaching. The client is obviously uncomfortable and will probably be unable to concentrate on or retain the information provided.

Example. James Boardman is a 56 year old who is receiving intravenous antibiotics for an infected wound. The medication is ordered every eight hours. When selecting administration times, the nurse chooses 6 A.M., 2 P.M., and 10 P.M. rather than 2 A.M., 10 A.M., and 6 P.M.

In this case, the nurse's choice avoids disruption of the client's sleep at 2 A.M. This allows Mr. Boardman to conserve the energy required for the healing process.

The nurse must also be sure to allow adequate time for completion of the nursing order. A thorough understanding of the actions necessary to implement the nursing order will allow the nurse to anticipate the time required. Careful organization will prevent the problems associated with hasty implementation.

Example. Kate Clinger is a community health nurse who is seeing a number of clients in a clinic. As she examines Jason Kovar, she discovers a serious skin irritation around his colostomy. Kate recognizes that the initiation of the measures required to manage the problem will involve a great deal of time. Therefore, she asks another nurse to see the waiting clients so that she can adequately treat Mr. Kovar's skin problem.

Personnel

The nurse should ensure the availability of sufficient numbers of personnel to implement the intervention.

Example. Henry Smithson is a 27 year old athlete who is recovering from chest surgery for a pneumothorax. He is six ft tall and weighs 255 lb. In preparing to ambulate this client for the first time, the nurse anticipates the need for assistance by at least one additional staff member. This will prevent injury to the client or nurse during the ambulation process.

Equipment

Another consideration when preparing to implement nursing interventions is the identification and procurement of necessary supplies. Again, the nurse must have a thorough understanding of the identified nursing action. This allows the anticipation of required equipment.

Example. In preparing to assist with the insertion of a urethral catheter, the nurse recognizes that a variety of equipment is required. These supplies include a light, a drape, a catheter, a drainage bag, lubricant, cotton balls, and antiseptic solution.

The nurse's inability to anticipate the need for the equipment in this case may predispose the client to infection. Therefore, the nurse should determine and provide the supplies necessary to ensure that the intervention is accomplished in an efficient and timely fashion.

Preparing a Conducive Environment

Successful implementation of nursing actions requires an environment in which the client feels comfortable and safe. Chapter 2 described a number of approaches designed to create a therapeutic environment in which clients can work toward resolving the factors that are contributing to the presence of problems.

Comfort

The creation of a comfortable environment involves consideration of both physical and psychosocial components. Physical concerns include the immediate environment (e.g., room, space, etc.), privacy, noise, odor, lighting, and temperature.

Example. Ed Kearney is a 78 year old man who had a cataract extraction three days ago. Following discharge from the hospital, he is being managed by his family at home with the assistance of a visiting nurse. Mr. Kearney requires a daily change of his eye patch and administration of medication. Before removal of the dressing, the nurse ensures that the shades are pulled and the room darkened to avoid the pain associated with exposure to light.

The nurse must also consider psychosocial concerns when preparing to implement nursing actions. These frequently require the use of interpersonal skills to provide an environment in which clients are comfortable in expressing their needs, fears, feelings, concerns, and frustrations. This usually involves both verbal and nonverbal communication skills, including interviewing, counseling, listening, and demonstrating.

Safety

A number of factors must be considered when the nurse attempts to create a safe environment. These include the client's age, degree of mobility, sensory deficits, and level of consciousness or orientation.

Age. When considering age, certainly the very young and the elderly are at greatest risk of injury. However, any environment that is unfamiliar to the client may be hazardous.

The infant and the toddler may be unable to communicate sensations such as pain or burning. Additionally, young children tend to explore their environment and the objects in it. Therefore, the nurse, in preparing to initiate procedures, must ensure that special consideration is given to the child's safety.

Example. Kevin Chen is a four year old admitted to pediatrics with a diagnosis of insulin-dependent diabetes. Kevin requires intravenous therapy and frequent insulin injections.

In managing Kevin's care, the nurse is careful to ensure that his IV line is securely taped to reduce the possibility that he will pull it out. The control clamp is also placed out of Kevin's reach to prevent him from inadvertently increasing the infusion rate. When preparing to administer injections, the nurse also checks type and dosage carefully and secures assistance if necessary to prevent injury at the time of injection.

Developmental changes associated with aging also require that the nurse prepare a safe environment for the elderly client. Decreased muscle strength and reflex speed prevent the older individual from recovering lost balance. Aging may also be accompanied by decreased visual and hearing acuity.

Degree of Mobility. The client's degree of mobility may be affected by disease or trauma, external restrictions such as traction or casts, or the need to conserve energy or equilibrium.

Example. John Cambria is a 28 year old man admitted to the hospital for lumbar strain. His physician has ordered bedrest, with bathroom privileges for BM only.

In anticipating the care of Mr. Cambria, the nurse is careful to place necessary supplies, such as water and the call bell, within his reach. This helps the client to avoid moving or reaching incorrectly and reduces the potential for further back strain. The nurse also instructs him to call for assistance when getting out of bed to avoid the potential for injury associated with a sudden drop in blood pressure after long periods of bedrest.

Sensory Deficits. The client who has decreased perception in sight, hearing, smell, taste, or touch may be at risk for injury. The nurse may be required to adapt the environment to protect the client's safety.

Example. Gladys Goldstein is a 26 year old quadraplegic who has developed an inflammation on her left thigh. She is seen in the outpatient clinic by a nurse practitioner. Orders include continuous warm soaks to her left thigh.

In this case, because Gladys has no feeling in her lower extremities, the nurse will attempt to ensure that the hazards of the treatment are reduced. This may be accomplished by instructing Gladys and her husband to check the temperature of the solutions and to inspect her skin frequently for evidence of burns.

Example. Sadie Bush is an 89 year old client who has been blind for ten years as a result of glaucoma. She is being admitted to a nursing home because she is no longer capable of caring for herself.

The nurse who admits Sadie may spend a great deal of time orienting her to this new environment and rearranging furniture to minimize the possibility that Sadie may be injured.

Clients with less serious visual deficits may be encouraged to wear corrective lenses. The nurse should also remind the client with a hearing deficit to wear a hearing aid if available. In addition, the nurse may touch the client to attract attention, approach from the client's good side, or allow the client to see the nurse before attempting to communicate or initiate other interventions.

Level of Consciousness/Orientation. Clients who have decreased levels of consciousness or are disoriented often require special attention or interventions to promote safety. Clients may be lethargic, stuporous, confused, or disoriented. These responses require the nurse to adjust the environment to prevent injury.

Example. Tyrone Magee is a 54 year old man who is recovering from a cerebral concussion. He is frequently disoriented and is found wandering in the hall looking for his dog.

The nurse who is managing Mr. Magee's care reorients him and returns him to his room. In addition, she puts the bed in the lowest position, arranges the room so that he will not fall, and keeps a light on in his room at night.

The care of an unconscious client may require similar adaptations.

Example. Al Rogers, age 62, is comatose following a massive CVA (stroke). He is restless at times and has had many seizures in the last 24 hours.

In this situation, the nurse may initiate a number of measures to protect the client. They may include padding the side rails, frequent changes in position, special skin care, and passive range of motion exercises.

Identifying Legal and Ethical Concerns

In preparing to implement nursing actions, the nurse must consider three areas: (1) client's rights, (2) nursing ethics, and (3) legal issues.

Client's Rights

In 1973, the American Hospital Association (AHA) published a bill of rights for the health care consumer (Figure 7–1). The purpose of the bill was to improve the quality of care and increase client satisfaction. Basically, the bill recognized the client's right to

□ considerate and respectful care
□ obtain information from the physician
□ informed consent
□ refuse treatment
□ privacy
□ confidentiality
□ reasonable response to requests
□ information regarding relationships among institutions or professionals involved in treatment
□ knowledge about research
□ continuity of care
□ information and explanation regarding bills
□ rules and regulations regarding clients' conduct

A PATIENT'S BILL OF RIGHTS

The American Hospital Association presents a Patient's Bill of Rights with the expectation that observance of these rights will contribute to more effective patient care and greater satisfaction for the patient, his physician, and the hospital organization. Further, the Association presents these rights in the expectation that they will be supported by the hospital on behalf of its patients, as an integral part of the healing process. It is recognized that a personal relationship between the physician and the patient is essential for the provision of proper medical care. The traditional physician-patient relationship takes on a new dimension when care is rendered within an organizational structure. Legal precedent has established that the institution itself also has a responsibility to the patient. It is in recognition of these factors that these rights are affirmed.

1. The patient has the right to considerate and respectful care.

2. The patient has the right to obtain from his physician complete current information concerning his diagnosis, treatment, and prognosis in terms the patient can be reasonably expected to understand. When it is not medically advisable to give such information to the patient, the information should be made available to an appropriate person in his behalf. He has the right to know, by name, the physician responsible for coordinating his care.

3. The patient has the right to receive from his physician information necessary to give informed consent prior to the start of any procedure and/or treatment. Except in emergencies, such information for informed consent should include but not necessarily be limited to the specific procedure and/or treatment, the medically significant risks involved, and the probable duration of incapacitation. Where medically significant alternatives for care or treatment exist, or when the patient requests information concerning medical alternatives, the patient has the right to such information. The patient also has the right to know the name of the person responsible for the procedures and/or treatment.

4. The patient has the right to refuse treatment to the extent permitted by law and to be informed of the medical consequences of his action.

5. The patient has the right to every consideration of his privacy concerning his own medical care program. Case discussion, consultation, examination, and treatment are confidential and should be conducted discreetly. Those not directly involved in his care must have the permission of the patient to be present.

6. The patient has the right to expect that all communications and records pertaining to his care should be treated as confidential.

7. The patient has the right to expect that within its capacity a hospital must make reasonable response to the request of a patient for services. The hospital must provide evaluation, service, and/or referral as indicated by the urgency of the case. When medically permissible a patient may be transferred to another facility only after he has received complete information and explanation concerning the needs for and alternatives to such a transfer. The institution to which the patient is to be transferred must first have accepted the patient for transfer.

8. The patient has the right to obtain information as to any relationship of his hospital to other health care and educational institutions insofar as his care is concerned. The patient has the right to obtain information as to the existence of any professional relationships among individuals, by name, who are treating him.

9. The patient has the right to be advised if the hospital proposes to engage in or perform human experimentation affecting his care or treatment. The patient has the right to refuse to participate in such research projects.

10. The patient has the right to expect reasonable continuity of care. He has the right to know in advance what appointment times and physicians are available and where. The patient has the right to expect that the hospital will provide a mechanism whereby he is informed by his physician or a delegate of the physician of the patient's continuing health care requirements following discharge.

11. The patient has the right to examine and receive an explanation of his bill regardless of source of payment.

12. The patient has the right to know what hospital rules and regulations apply to his conduct as a patient.

Figure 7–1 □ A patient's bill of rights. (Reprinted with the permission of the American Hospital Association. Copyright 1972.)

Illustration continued on following page

No catalogue of rights can guarantee for the patient the kind of treatment he has a right to expect. A hospital has many functions to perform, including the prevention and treatment of disease, the education of both health professionals and patients, and the conduct of clinical research. All these activities must be conducted with an overriding concern for the patient and, above all, the recognition of his dignity as a human being. Success in achieving this recognition assures success in the defense of the rights of the patient.

Figure 7–1 □ *Continued*

The entire health team, including the nurse, needs to ensure that none of these rights are violated.

In a previously cited example, a client required periodic catheterization following a hysterectomy. When preparing the client for the procedure, the nurse must be sure to explain the procedure to the client, obtain consent, and provide privacy. Following insertion, the nurse should make the client aware of any special care required following the procedure. The client also has the right to refuse treatment.

Example. Lynne Capik is three days post-op following a cesarean section. She is receiving 3000 ml of intravenous fluids daily. Following an infiltration in her right arm, the nurse prepares to restart the infusion in her left arm. After explaining the rationale and procedure for reinsertion, Lynne refuses to have the infusion restarted. She indicates that she wishes to discuss this with her physician.

In this instance, the client has the right to refuse such treatment, particularly after adequate information has been provided.

Nursing Ethics

Ethics has been defined as "the free rational assessment of courses of action in relation to principles, rules, conduct" (Churchill, 1977). There are a number of codes that define ethical principles. The ANA Code for Nurses (Figure 7–2) is a guideline that identifies the nurse's responsibility to consider ethical dilemmas associated with the nursing process. Additionally, the code defines the nurse's accountability for the decisions made regarding the client's welfare.

Ethical decision-making is often associated with the client's rights to informed consent, refusal of treatment, considerate treatment, and privacy. The nurse is commonly the liaison between the client and other health practitioners. This position often requires the nurse to advocate the client's position.

Example. Deborah Capone's breast biopsy reveals a cancerous tumor in her right breast. The physician has scheduled the client for a radical

---

AMERICAN NURSES' ASSOCIATION CODE FOR NURSES

1. The nurse provides services with respect for human dignity and the uniqueness of the client unrestricted by considerations of social or economic status, personal attributes, or the nature of health problems.

2. The nurse safeguards the client's right to privacy by judiciously protecting information of a confidential nature.

3. The nurse acts to safeguard the client and the public when health care and safety are affected by incompetent, unethical, or illegal practice of any person.

4. The nurse assumes responsibility and accountability for individual nursing judgments and actions.

5. The nurse maintains competence in nursing.

6. The nurse exercises informed judgment and uses individual competence and qualifications as criteria in seeking consultation, accepting responsibilities, and delegating nursing activities to others.

7. The nurse participates in activities that contribute to the ongoing development of the profession's body of knowledge.

8. The nurse participates in the profession's efforts to implement and improve standards of nursing.

9. The nurse participates in the profession's efforts to establish and maintain conditions of employment conducive to high quality nursing care.

10. The nurse participates in the profession's effort to protect the public from misinformation and misrepresentation and to maintain the integrity of nursing.

11. The nurse collaborates with members of the health professions and other citizens in promoting community and national efforts to meet the health needs of the public.

Figure 7–2 □ American Nurses' Association Code for Nurses.

mastectomy. The evening before surgery, the client indicates that she does not want to have the surgery. She questions, "Don't I have the right to get another opinion?"

In this case, the nurse has an ethical obligation to make the physician aware of the client's feelings. Additionally, the client's request for another opinion should be supported.

Nurses must be careful to avoid violations of the client's rights to privacy and confidentiality. When preparing to initiate nursing actions, the nurse should ensure that the client is not exposed and that sensitive discussions are not conducted inappropriately. Discussion of the client's diagnosis, prognosis, or problems should be conducted in a professional manner. These areas should not be topics of conversation over lunch or within earshot of visitors or other clients.

Legal Issues

Nurses are required to maintain a standard of care when implementing nursing actions. This is the "degree of care exercised by nurses of similar training or experience" (Cazalas, 1978). Violation of the standard of care may involve negligence on the nurse's part. Four basic elements must be present to substantiate negligence.

1. Duty to the client—the nurse has an obligation to manage the client using reasonable care (as defined by the standards of care).

2. Breach of the duty—this indicates that the duty to the client was violated.

3. Injury—the client must have incurred physical or emotional damage.

4. The injury must be a result of the breach of duty.

Negligence may include acts of omission, such as failure to initiate a medication or treatment that has been ordered by the physician. It may also include acts of commission, such as performing the treatment or giving the medication to the wrong client.

Example. In the implementation of intravenous therapy, the nurse is responsible for observing the site for redness, swelling, or drainage. In the event that these are present, the nurse should stop the infusion and restart it in another site (duty to the client). If the nurse fails to observe the site or fails to stop the intravenous infusion, this may be considered a breach of duty to the client. Subsequently, the client experiences painful inflammation and tissue sloughing at the site (injury sustained as a result of the breach of duty).

The nurse may also be negligent in delegating responsibility to other health practitioners.

Example. Suppose a registered nurse directs a licensed practical nurse to perform a nursing function that the latter is not qualified to carry out. Assume that the licensed practical nurse follows the order without question and harm occurs to the client; and assume that the registered nurse knows or should have known that the licensed practical nurse is not qualified (Hemelt and Mackert, 1982).

In this case, both parties would be negligent. The registered nurse would be liable for delegating a responsibility not normally expected of an LPN. The RN has a duty to assign appropriate personnel (duty), that responsibility is violated (breach of duty), and as a result, the client is harmed (injury as a result of breach of duty). The LPN has the responsibility to know personal qualifications and limitatations and would be liable for performing a procedure without proper qualifications.

Other areas of legal concern include assault and battery, false imprisonment, invasion of privacy, and defamation of character. Battery is the intentional touching of another without consent, and assault is the suggestion or threat of battery (Cazalas, 1978). If a patient refuses a treatment and the nurse indicates that it will be done anyway, assault has occurred. If the nurse actually performs the procedure, it would be battery.

False imprisonment is the conscious restraint of the freedom of another individual without the proper authorization, privilege, or consent of the individual (Hemelt and Mackert, 1982). An example of false imprisonment would occur if the nurse improperly restrained a client. However, if the client is a danger to self or others, restraint without consent would be accepable.

Invasion of privacy occurs when information given in confidence is released without the knowledge or consent of the client (Murray, 1980). This most commonly occurs in health care settings with the management of the client's medical record. The sharing of information on the client's chart should be limited to those directly involved in the care of the client.

Defamation of character is a communication about another person that exposes the person to contempt or diminishes his or her reputation. When written, defamation is termed *libel*. Oral defamation is termed *slander* (Hemelt and Mackert, 1982). The inclusion of false or injurious information on the client's medical record is an example of libel. Discussion of this same information with other clients or health care workers is slander.

Medical records are frequently utilized in resolving legal issues. Therefore, the importance of accurate and thorough documentation cannot be overemphasized. The record reflects the care provided to the client and as such may be utilized as defense in a legal proceeding.

STAGE II—INTERVENTION

The focus of the implementation phase is the initiation of nursing orders designed to meet the client's physical or emotional needs. The nurse's approach may involve the initiation of independent, dependent, and interdependent actions. The approaches designed to meet the client's physical and emotional needs are numerous and varied, depending on individual, specific problems. However, there are some common components involved in the implementation of nursing interventions. These factors include continuous assessment, planning, and teaching.

The initial detailed assessment was covered in Chapter 2. The assessment process utilized during the implementation phase is ongoing and involves the nurse's ability to collect and process data before, during, and after the initiation of nursing interventions. For example, before getting a postoperative client out of bed, the nurse observes that he is short of breath and slightly diaphoretic. Based on these findings, the nurse assesses the client's vital signs and chooses to defer his ambulation at that time. On the basis of the data obtained from the ongoing assessment, the nurse decides whether to initiate, continue, modify, or discontinue individual nursing orders.

During the implementation process, the planning component is also continuous. The nurse may be required to revise or discontinue an order based on client response or assessment findings. For example, while performing ostomy care, the nurse determines that, because of the placement of the stoma, it is difficult to achieve adherence of the client's pouch using the standard equipment. At that point, the nurse decides to use an alternate pouch that will ensure a good seal and protect the client's skin. The nurse does not wait until the entire plan of care is changed to implement an alternative approach. This reflects the ongoing planning process during implementation.

Teaching is often a formal component of the care plan, as demonstrated in Chapter 6. However, the structured teaching plan is only one approach used by the nurse. Informal teaching is frequently incorporated into the implementation process. During the process of providing care, the nurse may describe what happens during a radiology or laboratory procedure, how a catheter works, or why it is important to check the pulse before taking certain medications. This type of teaching, although less formal in nature, allows the nurse to respond to the client's immediate needs or questions. This facilitates positive nurse-client relationships and ensures the delivery of a higher quality of care.

The client's physical and emotional needs are identified in the assessment phase of the nursing process. A nursing diagnosis and outcomes are formulated, and individualized nursing orders are written. During the implementation phase, the nurse initiates these interventions. The following subsections discuss the type of interventions used based on the 11 functional health patterns identified by Gordon (1982). Table 7–1 divides the patterns into physical or emotional categories. A definition and description are provided for each pattern. Commonly associated nursing diagnoses are listed based on the work of Gordon (1982) and Carpenito (1983). Additionally, contributing factors are identified for each pattern. The focus for interventions in each area is presented, along with sample methods of implementation. Note that each pattern frequently requires the initiation of assessment, planning, and teaching.

TABLE 7–1 □ **CATEGORIES OF FUNCTIONAL HEALTH PATTERNS**

Physical	Emotional
Health perception–health management	Self-perception–self-concept
Nutritional-metabolic	Role-relationship
Elimination	Sexuality-reproductive
Activity-exercise	Coping–stress tolerance
Sleep-rest	Value-belief
Cognitive-perceptual	

Physical Patterns

Those patterns identified as physical include health perception–health management, nutritional-metabolic, elimination, activity-exercise, sleep-rest, and cognitive-perceptual. The following will define and describe each pattern, identify associated nursing diagnoses, and describe nursing interventions.

Health Perception–Health Management

Definition. This pattern describes individual, family, or community perceptions of health and defines the usual practices utilized to promote or maintain health. This identification assists the nurse to develop nursing orders that are (1) consistent with positive health practices, (2) designed to clarify the client's incorrect perceptions, and (3) directed toward identification of alternative health strategies.

Associated Nursing Diagnoses	Contributing Factors
1. Alterations in health maintenance	Lack of knowledge, existing unhealthy lifestyle, inacessibility to necessary resources, anxiety, nontherapeutic relationships or environment, physical or perceptual deficits, age, changes in self-image
2. Noncompliance	
3. Potential for injury	

Interventions. The implementation of nursing interventions may be directed toward (1) identification of unhealthy patterns through assessment or screening, (2) provision of health education, including formal and informal teaching approaches involving the client, family, or community at large, (3) identification of available resources, including personnel, finances, and equipment, and (4) initiation of environmental changes, if required.

Example. Al Rogers, a 42 year old man, is seen in his physician's office with a diagnosis of urinary tract infection. In assessing this client's perception of health, the nurse identifies that he considers himself to be basically healthy and feels that this problem can be managed effectively by careful attention to prescribed orders, minor lifestyle changes, and regular follow-up.

In this case, the nurse's approach will include reinforcement of the client's positive perceptions and careful explanation of therapeutic approaches.

Example. Pat O'Brien, age 42, is admitted to a same day surgery unit for a biopsy of her left breast. The nurse's assessment indicates that the client's mother died eight years ago from metastatic breast cancer. The nurse also determines that Pat does not perform breast self-examination or have regular gynecological check-ups.

The nurse's interventions in this case will focus on identifying the risk factors associated with malignant breast disease, particularly age and familial history. Additionally, the nurse must communicate the need for regular preventive approaches.

Nutritional-Metabolic

Definition. This describes the client's usual pattern of consumption of food or fluids. The client's status is based on the identification of metabolic need and a subsequent comparison of the client's food and fluid intake as well as nutritional supplements, height, weight, skin, and mucous membranes. This allows the nurse (1) to identify incorrect perceptions regarding food and fluid consumption, (2) to anticipate potential problems, and (3) to determine definitive approaches to prevent or correct them.

Associated Nursing Diagnoses	Contributing Factors
1. Fluid volume deficit 2. Fluid volume excess 3. Alteration in nutrition: less than body requirements 4. Alteration in nutrition: more than body requirements 5. Alteration in oral mucous membrane 6. Impaired skin integrity	Elevated temperature, burns, irritating or excessive drainage, infection, nausea or vomiting, nasogastric suction, anorexia, blood loss, weakness, effects of therapy, diarrhea, excessive sodium intake, immobility, swallowing difficulties, wired jaw, lack of knowledge, loneliness, boredom, sedentary lifestyle, inadequate oral hygiene

Interventions. Nursing interventions will be directed toward (1) identification of specific unhealthy patterns, (2) determination of the factors precipitating their potential or actual occurrence, (3) initiation of specific approaches to prevent or correct individual nutritional problems, (4) provision of specific education, when required, and (5) identification of available resources.

Example. Carla Ramirez is seen for the first time in a prenatal clinic. She is 17 years old and is pregnant with her second child. Her first baby was delivered two months prematurely and died three days after birth. Carla indicates that she is unmarried and on welfare and lives with her parents and nine siblings.

The nurse identifies that this client has specific nutritional needs because of her pregnancy. Assessment also indicates a number of factors that will interfere with the client's ability to satisfy these needs. Therefore, the nurse will implement orders designed to increase the potential for Carla to obtain the food, milk, and vitamin supplements required during pregnancy.

Example. Glenn Stevens, age 86, is admitted with a fractured humerus, which requires skeletal traction. The nurse identifies that Mr. Stevens is thin and slightly dehydrated and has limited mobility as a result of the continuous traction.

In this case, the nurse recognizes that the client's decreased nutritional and fluid status in combination with static positioning exposes him to the potential for altered skin integrity. The nurse's approach would include nutritional supplementation, increased fluid intake, and skin protection measures.

Elimination

Definition. This pattern describes the client's ability to eliminate body wastes, including those of bowel and bladder. Critical indicators focus on regularity and control. The nurse evaluates usual patterns of bowel and bladder elimination, including the existence of alternative routes (e.g., ostomy). This allows the nurse (1) to identify incorrect perceptions related to bowel or bladder function, (2) to anticipate actual or potential deficits, (3) to propose alternative approaches to facilitate elimination or correct known deficits, and (4) to assess the effects of existing deviations.

Associated Nursing Diagnoses	Contributing Factors
1. Alteration in bowel elimination: constipation, diarrhea, incontinence 2. Alteration in urinary elimination: enuresis, dysuria, incontinence	Immobility, effects of therapy, pregnancy, pain, lack of privacy, decreased fluid intake, stress, lack of knowledge, use of laxatives, irritating foods, tube feedings, dehydration, infection, diminished bladder capacity, barriers to ambulation

Interventions. The implementation of nursing approaches may be directed toward (1) defining normal elimination patterns and comparing them with current patterns, (2) identifying specific contributing factors, (3) developing preventive or corrective approaches to ensure positive elimination, and (4) providing education as required.

Example. James Balfour is a 49 year old man admitted for cervical strain. His treatment modality includes bedrest, moist heat, ultrasound therapy, and the use of analgesics (acetaminophen [Tylenol] with codeine). Mr. Balfour identifies that he is constipated and expresses concern to the nurse.

The nurse recognizes that the treatment regimen required to manage Mr. Balfour's back problem predisposes him to bowel elimination problems. This is the result of a combination of immobility and the effects of codeine. The nurse implements interventions designed to reduce or eliminate this problem, which include providing adequate roughage in his diet, increasing fluid intake, and suggesting the need for stool softeners.

Example. Joan Terrence is seen in the community health clinic for follow-up after a temporary colostomy for diverticulitis. The client indicates that her ostomy functions regularly every other day, and the nurse finds that the condition of her stoma and skin is excellent.

Although this client's method of elimination is altered, the nurse is able to assess that the client perceives her ostomy to be functioning normally. Additionally, the nurse determines that the client's normal pattern of elimination has resumed. Therefore, the interventions in this case will focus on reinforcing the client's perceptions and providing additional resources as required.

Activity-Exercise

Definition. This pattern includes a broad range of concerns that focus on specific activities requiring the expenditure of energy. These consist of the common activities of daily living, such as eating, hygiene, grooming, and toileting, as well as leisure and recreation. Critical indicators also include mobility and respiratory and cardiac functions, since alterations in these areas may predispose the client to activity and exercise problems.

Associated Nursing Diagnoses	Contributing Factors
1. Activity intolerance	Prolonged immobility, pain, fa-
2. Ineffective airway clearance	tigue, effects of therapy, retained
3. Ineffective breathing patterns	secretions, weakness, decreased

4. Decreased cardiac output
5. Diversional activity deficit
6. Impaired gas exchange
7. Impaired home maintenance management
8. Impaired physical mobility
9. Self-care deficit
10. Alteration in tissue perfusion

oxygenation, depression, sedentary lifestyle, effects of surgery, lack of motivation, smoking, high-risk environment, fear, absent or nonfunctioning body parts, presence of invasive lines, hypothermia, infection, inadequate nutritional intake, decreased physical activity, lack of knowledge, limited range of motion

Interventions. The implementation of nursing approaches may be directed toward (1) identifying usual activity-exercise patterns, (2) evaluating client responses to activity based on findings, (3) implementing preventive, supportive, or therapeutic approaches to minimize effects on lifestyle, and (4) providing client and family education as required.

Example. Carlton Henning is a 58 year old man with metastatic cancer of the lung who is being followed at home by the visiting nurse. As a result of his disease process, Mr. Henning's activity is restricted to bedrest at this time. In addition, he is home alone a large amount of the time, since his wife must work to support the family. The nurse often observes the client looking out of the window and staring for prolonged periods of time.

Mr. Henning obviously has a number of problems of concern. His mobility and respiratory functions are impaired, and his activity tolerance is limited. In this case, the nurse may also focus on the provision of diversional activities designed to alter his limited routine. These could include reading, playing cards, watching television, or listening to classical music.

Example. Cathy Sizemore is a 37 year old woman admitted to the hospital with advanced multiple sclerosis. She is divorced and lives with her elderly mother, who has chronic congestive heart failure. With the progression of her disease, Cathy is now confined to a wheelchair and verbalizes concern about her ability to manage the upkeep of her apartment.

Here, the nurse recognizes that an active diagnosis of impaired home maintenance management exists. At this point, the nurse will explore available resources to assist Cathy and her mother in their present living situation. Subsequently, it may be necessary to discuss long-term arrangements in alternative settings, should they be required.

Sleep-Rest

Definition. This pattern focuses on the client's ability to obtain sleep, rest, or relaxation. The nurse attempts to define the client's normal sleep patterns and their subsequent effects on the activities of daily living. Critical factors include identification of sleep requirements, additional restful activities, and the client's ability to implement relaxation techniques when appropriate.

Associated Nursing Diagnosis	Contributing Factors
Sleep pattern disturbance	Pain, anxiety, impaired elimination, hospitalization, effects of therapy, pregnancy, depression, stress, unfamiliar environment

Interventions. The implementation of nursing approaches may be directed toward (1) identifying the client's normal sleep-rest pattern, (2) determining the client's perception of the effects of the usual pattern, (3) initiating measures to increase the duration or quality of sleep and rest, (4) promoting relaxation through physical or mental techniques, and (5) providing health teaching for the client and family as necessary.

Example. Ken Slater is a truck driver who is hospitalized for surgery to repair an inguinal hernia. He is frequently observed walking in the hall or watching television during the night. However, he sleeps at long intervals during the day.

The nurse's initial assessment of this client's behavior suggests a sleep pattern disturbance. However, further discussion with the client reveals that he usually drives for long periods at night when traffic is lighter and sleeps during the day. Therefore, the nurse would attempt to maintain his normal pattern and provide frequent rest periods during the day.

Example. Andrew Hardy is a 52 year old man admitted to the hospital with recurrent angina. He has been pain-free for two days. However, he is unable to sleep for longer than a two-hour interval. The client indicates that he usually sleeps about six hours nightly. Mr. Hardy states that he is concerned about losing his job, since this is his third hospitalization this year.

In this case, the nurse recognizes both short- and long-term sleep-rest implications. The initiation of relaxation techniques may be utilized immediately to increase the duration of the client's sleep pattern. Additionally, the nurse should incorporate health teaching strategies, including stress management to alleviate usual job demands.

Cognitive-Perceptual

Definition. This pattern describes the client's sensory abilities (hearing, seeing, taste, smell, and touch) as well as higher level cognitive functions (language, memory, decision-making, problem solving). The nurse attempts to identify usual patterns, specific deficits, and compensatory mechanisms utilized by the client.

Associated Nursing Diagnoses	Contributing Factors
1. Alteration in comfort 2. Knowledge deficit 3. Sensory-perceptual alterations 4. Alterations in thought processes	Pain, effects of surgery, anxiety, social or cultural barriers, ineffective coping patterns, age, unfamiliar environment, effects of therapy, substance abuse, immobility, pregnancy, sensory overload or deprivation, isolation, fear, depression, conflict

Interventions. The implementation of nursing approaches may be directed toward (1) determining the source of the client's deficits in sensation or perception, (2) identifying positive mechanisms currently utilized as well as other potential approaches, (3) providing specific education regarding temporary measures and long-term potential for managing problems, and (4) obtaining additional resources when required.

Example. Nina Tallone had a stroke five days ago. The nurse notes that she has difficulty in expressing her thoughts and short-term memory losses. As a result, Mrs. Tallone is hesitant to respond to questioning or to participate in conversations with unfamiliar people. She is also frustrated by her inability to recall recent events.

The nurse's approach to the management of this client's problems may focus on educating her about the disease process and effects of stroke. Additional strategies for managing memory loss and utilization of approaches suggested by a speech therapist may be of value.

Example. Tom Gorski is a policeman who is being seen in the physician's office for persistent hypertension. The nurse's interactions with this client reveal a total lack of knowledge regarding the disease process, the need for frequent monitoring, the effects of high salt intake, and the relationship between stress and the occurrence of hypertension.

Here, the nurse's action is clearly defined—the development and implementation of a comprehensive teaching plan. Consideration must be given to incorporating some of the client's usual patterns to ensure compliance with the prescribed strategies.

Emotional Patterns

Those patterns identified as a reflection of the emotional component of the client's needs are self-perception, role-relationship, sexuality-reproductive, coping–stress tolerance, and value-belief.

Self-Perception

Definition. This pattern defines the client's perception of self in terms of four predominant variables—body image, self-esteem, role performance, and personal identity (Carpenito, 1983). The nurse attempts to identify the effects of change, loss, or threat on the client's self-perception.

Associated Nursing Diagnoses	Contributing Factors
1. Anxiety 2. Fear 3. Powerlessness 4. Disturbance in self-concept	Feelings of helplessness, change, actual or perceived threat, loss of body part or function, hospitalization, terminal disease, disability, effects of therapy, pain, lack of knowledge, inadequate coping, loss of job, divorce, pregnancy, stress

Interventions. The implementation of nursing approaches may be directed toward (1) assisting the client to define perception of self and its relationship to health, (2) identifying specific variables contributing to the client's problems, (3) assisting the client to develop problem-solving skills to deal with the effects of change, loss, or threat, and (4) providing education or referral to additional resources when required.

Example. JoEllen Parker is a 12 year old girl who visits the school nurse's office frequently with vague somatic complaints. The nurse's approach has been to investigate each complaint and to reassure JoEllen. During these conversations, the nurse learns that this client feels awkward because she is about 5 inches taller than all of her friends, including the boys in class. She also has begun to menstruate and is afraid that others will find out and make fun of her.

The nurse recognizes that this client's self-image has been affected by rapid body changes associated with puberty. Nursing approaches will focus on continuing their trusting relationship and assisting JoEllen to deal with rapid physical changes compounded by peer pressure.

Example. Frank Nicholas is an elderly client who is transferred from the coronary care unit following a myocardial infarction (heart attack) complicated by heart failure. The nurse notes that he is apathetic and depressed and refuses to make decisions regarding his care. Eventually, the client reveals that he feels frustrated by the lack of information provided by his physician. He also indicates that "It doesn't matter what I think—they'll do what they want anyway."

This client is exhibiting behaviors that are typical of one who feels powerless in a health care setting. The nurse's role here is that of client-advocate. Interventions will focus on improving communication, educating the client about his rights in the health care system, and determining strategies to increase his degree of control over this situation.

Role-Relationship

Definition. This pattern describes the client's individual, family, and social roles. The client's perceptions of roles and relationships are important because they form a component of identity. Individuals require a variety of roles and levels of relationships to be self-actualized. The client's degree of satisfaction with roles and relationships and the level of independence attained are also important considerations.

Associated Nursing Diagnoses	Contributing Factors
1. Impaired verbal communication	Language barrier, aphasia, de-
2. Alterations in family processes	creased level of consciousness, in-
3. Grieving	tubation, pain, lack of privacy, ill-
4. Alterations in parenting	ness or loss of family member,
5. Social isolation	financial crisis, lack of support sys-
6. Potential for violence	tems, loss of function or body part,
	hospitalization, divorce, lack of
	knowledge, impaired bonding,
	stress, suicidal tendencies, anger,
	fear, drug or alcohol abuse

Interventions. The implementation of nursing approaches may be directed toward (1) assisting the client to identify individual, family, or social roles that are of concern, (2) examining the associated relationships to identify supporting or distressing features, (3) providing education or additional resources when necessary, and (4) assisting the client to develop strategies for managing those areas that are unsatisfying or undesirable.

Example. Lucy Caron is a 54 year old woman with a progressive neuro-muscular disease. Over a period of five months, she has had progressive paralysis, which resulted in respiratory problems requiring a tracheos-tomy. At this point, Mrs. Caron is unable to speak and has such limited movement in her left arm that she is unable to write. It is therefore extremely difficult for her to communicate with her family or the nursing staff.

In this case, the nurse recognizes the client's severe communication deficits. Therefore, the nurse requests the assistance of the occupational therapist. A computer is provided that allows the client to select a message that is printed on a screen for the family or staff. This enhances the client's personal and therapeutic relationships.

Example. Tony Angeli is a navy submarine officer who is frequently at sea for prolonged periods of time. Therefore, his interactions with his youngest son, age eight months, have been minimal. He verbalizes his frustration and feelings of parental failure in a conversation with the clinic nurse.

Here, the nurse's interventions focus on counseling to assist the father to achieve a more positive feeling about his parental role.

Sexuality-Reproductive

Definition. This pattern reflects the client's sexual identity and involves the client's ability to express sexuality and achieve satisfying individual or interpersonal relationships. This pattern also includes the status of the client's reproductive capabilities.

Associated Nursing Diagnoses	Contributing Factors
1. Sexual dysfunction 2. Rape trauma syndrome	Lack of knowledge, effects of therapy, hospitalization, loss of body part, unwilling partner, stress, lack of privacy, abuse, violent episode

Interventions. The implementation of nursing approaches may be directed toward (1) assisting the client to clarify individual perceptions related to sexuality and sexual identity, (2) identifying barriers to adequate sexual expression or feeling or to reproduction, (3) providing education regarding sexual or reproductive concerns, and (4) allowing the client to develop viable alternatives with nursing support.

Example. Chris Sopko is a 17 year old runaway seen in the community health clinic with symptoms of depression, withdrawal, and multiple sleep disturbances. He tells the nurse that he was raped by a male homosexual four months ago. He describes feelings of guilt and disgust and indicates that this was probably his punishment for running away.

The nurse's interventions in this case are directed toward providing psychological support to this traumatized client. The therapeutic relationship should be maintained, and the nurse should reassure the client, help him to resolve his guilt feelings, and assist him to develop a realistic plan for the future. Additional counseling or therapy may be recommended if necessary.

Example. Pam Bernhardt is a 52 year old client seen in the doctor's office six weeks following a hysterectomy. She verbalizes her concern about resuming sexual relations with her husband, indicating that "it just won't be the same."

In this example, the nurse utilizes a supportive approach, explains the normalcy of the client's response, and encourages open dialogue between the client and her spouse. Her fears may be unfounded, and in fact, their relationship may improve as a result of this type of dialogue.

Coping–Stress Tolerance

Definition. This pattern involves the identification of the types and degree of stress associated with the client's lifestyle. The coping mechanisms utilized by the individual and the family are identified as well as the client's ability to manage various levels of stress. The client's perception of these variables are particularly important in this pattern, because interventions must be directed to what the client perceives to be problematic.

Associated Nursing Diagnoses	Contributing Factors
1. Ineffective individual coping 2. Ineffective family coping	Loss of job, divorce, relocation, sensory overload or deprivation, persistent stress, loss of body part, feelings of helplessness, hospitalization, terminal illness, domestic violence

Interventions. The implementation of nursing interventions may be directed toward (1) assisting the client to identify personal patterns of response to individual or family stress, (2) identifying the sources of stress for the client as an individual, (3) developing positive coping strategies to avoid distress, (4) providing education regarding identified variables and the use of relaxation, and (5) obtaining additional resources when required.

Example. Ken Cord is an elderly client hospitalized in an intensive care unit as a result of respiratory failure secondary to chronic obstructive lung disease. He has been in the unit for three weeks and suddenly begins screaming that he can't take it anymore. He states that all the noises are "driving me crazy, I never get any rest, and I'm tired of all this fussing and these newfangled machines."

This is a classic response to the sensory overload associated with critical care areas. In this situation, the nurse utilizes interpersonal skills to assist the client to identify alternate coping strategies. The use of relaxation techniques may be particularly beneficial if accompanied by a reduction in environmental stimulation.

Example. Marilyn Holcombe, a 32 year old woman, is examined in the emergency department following a beating by her husband. Marilyn states that her husband becomes abusive when he drinks. "I'd like to leave him, but I'm afraid he'll find me," she says.

The nurse recognizes the need to assist Marilyn in coping with her husband's behavior. This may involve encouraging the client to discuss her feelings about this current situation, her desire for a change, and the availability of support systems.

Value-Belief

Definition. This pattern defines the client and family belief systems. These include what the client believes to be correct and valuable based on personal knowledge, individual and community norms, or faith. The client's perception of the value of preventive care, treatment modalities, or even life itself may influence individual ability to manage the problems associated with conflicting beliefs or value systems.

Associated Nursing Diagnosis	Contributing Factors
1. Spiritual distress	Hospitalization, conflicting value systems, inability to practice rituals, terminal disease, effects of therapy, isolation

Interventions. Nursing interventions will be directed toward (1) identifying the specific value or belief pattern involved, (2) determining particular sources of conflict, when appropriate, (3) obtaining available resources to facilitate the practice of religious beliefs or the resolution of conflicts, and (4) providing information regarding health management to assist the client in making informed choices regarding continued health practices.

Example. John and Carrie Davis are Jehovah's Witnesses. Their 16 year old daughter, Nancy, was involved in a sledding accident that resulted in a compound fracture of the ankle with bleeding into the joint. Mr. and Mrs. Davis oppose the use of blood transfusions on a religious basis and refuse to allow the administration of a transfusion during surgery.

The nurse recognizes the conflict between the parents' religious beliefs and their desire to save their child's life. In this case, the nurse ensures that the family is well-informed regarding alternative treatment modalities and possible adverse reactions. Additionally, the nurse supports the parents while they resolve this conflict.

STAGE III—DOCUMENTATION

The implementation of nursing orders must be followed by complete and accurate documentation of the events occurring in this stage of the nursing process. There are three types of systems of record-keeping utilized in the documentation of client care. They are (1) source-oriented records, (2) problem-oriented records, and (3) computer-assisted records. Each of these systems will be explored in this section.

Source-Oriented Records

The source-oriented system is the traditional charting system; it continues to be utilized by a number of institutions and agencies. In this system, information is recorded chronologically within specific time periods. The medical record is divided into sections according to the source of the data. Each discipline records information on a separate section—e.g., nurses' notes, physician progress notes, physical therapy notes, respiratory therapy notes, and social service notes.

The frequency of documentation in a source-oriented system is dependent upon the client's condition. In an acute care setting, notes may be documented as frequently as every few minutes for a critically ill client. More commonly, the nurse documents observations once each shift and includes assessment data, implementation of nursing and medical orders, and the client's response to nursing or medical interventions. In alternative settings, such as nursing homes, community health centers, or physicians' offices, findings may be documented less frequently—daily, weekly, monthly, or less often, as indicated by institutional policy or client contact.

The advantage of a source-oriented system is easy access to the location of the forms and subsequent documentation of each discipline. The disadvantages of this system include

□ Fragmentation of the documentation of the client's care according to the provider;
□ No clear definition of the client's problems or interdisciplinary approaches to manage them;
□ Lack of integrated documentation of the client's response to intervention;
□ Inconsistent documentation of teaching when accomplished by many disciplines—e.g., nursing, nutrition, respiratory therapy.
□ Greater difficulty in auditing the record when evaluating the quality of care delivered (Sorensen and Luckmann, 1979).

Samples of documentation in a source-oriented system are shown in Figures 7–3 and 7–4. Additional components of a source-oriented system may include flowsheets, graphic records, and the like. Flowsheets facilitate the systematic organization of information about the client. They may be utilized primarily for quick, efficient documentation of routine client care (Figure 7–5). Additionally, flowsheets may be valuable in identifying progression in terms of a number of parameters pertinent to the client's care (Figure 7–6).

Frequently, institutions and agencies utilizing source-oriented systems develop modifications to manage some of the difficulties associated with this method. The form seen in Figure 7–7 is utilized in combination with a flowsheet. The nurses' notes focus on active nursing diagnoses and include documentation of significant events that reflect the client's progress toward the outcomes outlined in the plan of care. The teaching record shown in Figure 7–8 demonstrates an organized approach to the implementation of an individualized teaching plan.

Problem-Oriented Records

The problem-oriented system of documentation parallels the nursing process. Each involves data collection, identification of client problems (nursing diagnoses), development and implementation of the plan of care, and evaluation of outcome achievement. In this system, information focuses on the client's problems (diagnoses) and is integrated and recorded by all disciplines, utilizing a consistent format. This facilitates multidisciplinary recording utilizing the same data base and progress notes. There-

Text continued on page 215

G-013

HAMILTON HOSPITAL

NURSES NOTES

(Patient Identifying Data)

DATE	HOUR	OBSERVATIONS AND REMARKS	SIGNATURE
12/27/85	7³⁰ AM	Client alert, oriented ᵃⁿᵈ responsive to verbal ᵃⁿᵈ tactile stimuli. No complaints of pain or discomfort at this time. I.V. infusing via #18 angio in left forearm. Hypoactive bowel sounds in R & L upper quadrants only. Breath sounds clear bilaterally. Coughing ᵃⁿᵈ deep breathing independently. Turns with minimal assistance	
	8⁰⁰ AM	Tolerated 450 cc clear liquids @ breakfast	
	8¹⁵ AM	Assisted with partial bath. I.V. dsgs. changed - no evidence of redness, swelling @ site. Anti-embolism stockings removed ᵃⁿᵈ reapplied. Abdominal dressing changed - no redness, swelling noted	
	8⁴⁵ AM	C/o incisional pain - medicated c̄ Demerol 100 mg. I.M.	
	9¹⁵ AM	Sleeping @ intervals with no C/o pain	
	11⁴⁵ AM	Foley catheter drained 300 cc clear amber urine - removed per M.D. order - encouraged to force fluids p.o.	
	12 noon	Tolerated 500 cc clear liquids for lunch - expelling flatus @ this time	
	1⁵⁰ pm	C/o incisional pain - medicated c̄ Demerol 100 mg. I.M	
	2¹⁵ pm	Voided 450 cc amber urine - C/o burning on urination - encouraged to continue forcing fluids	
	3⁰⁰ pm	Sleeping @ present	Janet M. York RN

Figure 7–3 □ Source note. (Courtesy of Hamilton Hospital, Trenton, NJ.)

PROGRESS NOTES

FAMILY NAME		FIRST NAME	ATTENDING PHYSICIAN	ROOM NO.	HOSPITAL NO.
DATE			Notes Should Be Signed By Physician		

8/20/85 9:45 AM — Initiated gait training on parallel bars. Stands well with encouragement but has some difficulty ambulating — unable to support self well because of cast on right forearm and hand. Instructed in alternate methods of stabilization. Able to walk length of parallel bars c̄ assistance x1 ——— Carol Merchiore RPT

Figure 7–4 □ Physical therapy source note. (Courtesy of Hamilton Hospital, Trenton, NJ.)

MEMORIAL HOSPITAL
OF BURLINGTON COUNTY

PATIENT CARE RECORD

DATE			11-7	7-3	3-11			11-7	7-3	3-11
HYGIENE	Self Care					SAFETY	Side rails up			
	Bedside						Restraint			
	Shower/Tub						Vest			
	Bath w/assistance						Wrist			
	Partial Bath						Ankle			
	Complete Bed Bath						Other			
	*Special Skin Care to Pressure Points						Released Q 2 hr			
	Back Rub					TREATMENTS	Oxygen Therapy			
	Foot Care						Mask I _____			
	Peri Care						Cannula I _____			
	Mouth Care						Egg Crate Mattress			
	H. S. Care						Surgical Stockings			
ACTIVITY	Unassisted						Removed 1 x /shift			
	Ambulatory w/assistance						Isolation Type _____			
	1-2 x /shift									
	3 or more x's/shift									
	Bedpan/Urinal w/assistance									
	1-2 x's/shift									
	3 or more x's/shift									
	Commode or BR w/assistance									
	1-2 x's/shift					SPECIAL TREATMENTS				
	3 or more x's/shift									
	Chair/Transfer w/assistance									
	1-2 x's/shift									
	3 or more x's/shift									
	Dangle w/assistance									
	Bedrest									
	Turns Self									
	Turn/Position w/assistance									
	1-2 x's/shift									
	3 or more x's/shift									
	Range of Motion									
NUTRITION	NPO									
	Self Feed									
	Feed w/assistance									
	Complete Feed									
	*Tube Feeding									
	Nasogastric									
	Gastrostomy									
	Intermittent									
	Continuous									
	Enteral Pump									
	Adequate Intake									
	*Inadequate Intake									
	Fluid Restriction Amt. _____									
	Force Fluids Amt. _____									
BOWEL	Stool Number									
	No Stool									
	Incontinent # x's									
BLADDER	Voiding Q S									
	Incontinent # x's									
	Foley Catheter									
SLEEP	Slept Well									
	Awake at Intervals									
	Awake Most of Time									

NURSES SIGNATURE AND STATUS & INITIALS

11-7 _____ Initials _____ Initials

7-3 _____ Initials _____ Initials

3-11 _____ Initials _____ Initials

NOTE: Document unusual or abnormal findings on Patient's Progress Record.

CODES:
* Further documentation required on Patient's Progress Record. Please initial in space as applicable.

070177 (3/85)

Figure 7–5 □ Patient care flowsheet. (Courtesy of Memorial Hospital of Burlington County, Mount Holly, NJ 08060.)

G-131 (Rev. 2/83)

HAMILTON HOSPITAL
NEUROLOGICAL NURSING ASSESSMENT

NURSES' INITIAL CODE								
Initial	Name			Status	Initial	Name		Status

DATE											
TIME											
INITIAL											
I. OPENS EYES (✓ Best Response)											
Spontaneously											
Opens to sound											
Opens to pain											
None											
II. BEST VERBAL RESPONSE (✓ Best Response)											
Oriented											
Confused											
Inappropriate words											
Incomprehensible sounds											
None											
III. BEST MOTOR RESPONSE (✓ Best Response)											
Moves spontaneously											
Obeys commands											
Flaccid											
IV. REFLEXES (mark + or −)											
Cough											
Gag											
Swallow											
Corneal											
Babinski											
CSF leak from nose											
CSF leak from ear											

Figure 7–6 □ Neurologic assessment flowsheet. (Courtesy of Hamilton Hospital, Trenton, NJ.)

Illustration continued on opposite page

DATE													
TIME													
INITIALS													
V. RESPONSES TO PAIN	R/L	R/L	R/L	R/L	R/L	R/L	R/L	R/L	R/L	R/L	R/L
UPPER EXTREMITIES (✓ Best Response)											
Localizes pain											
Withdraws											
Flexes											
Extends											
None											
LOWER EXTREMITIES (✓ Best Response)											
Localizes pain											
Withdraws											
Flexes											
Extends											
None											
VI. PUPILS (✓ Best Response) **SIZE**											
● Constricted											
◉ Normal											
◯ Dilated											
RESPONSE TO LIGHT (✓ Best Response)											
Brisk											
Sluggish											
No reaction											
Equal response											
Unequal response											
VII. PERIPHERAL PULSES (Mark + or −)											
Carotid											
Bracheal											
Radial											
Femoral											
Popliteal											
Dorsalis pedis											
Posterior tibialis											
VIII. SEIZURE ACTIVITY (+ or −)											
For description of seizure, please see nurses' notes											

Figure 7–6 □ *Continued*

G-013

HAMILTON HOSPITAL

NURSES NOTES

(Patient Identifying Data)

DATE/TIME	DIAGNOSIS	OBSERVATIONS AND REMARKS SIGNATURE
12/27/85 3:15 pm	Comfort	Client c/o incisional pain twice this shift. Medicated c̄ Demerol 100 mg IM @ 8:45 AM + 1:50 pm. Sleeping @ intervals after medication. Ice bag to incisional area
	Elimination (Urinary)	Foley catheter patent for 300cc clear amber urine - removed @ 11:45 AM per M.D. order. Voided 450 cc amber urine @ 2:15 pm - c/o burning when voiding - encouraged to force fluids - prefers apple juice to ginger ale.
	(bowel)	Hypoactive bowel sounds in R&L upper quadrants only - expelling flatus
	Nutrition	I.V. infusing via #18 angio in L forearm. Tolerating clear liquids by mouth - 1200 cc this shift
	S.N.N	Coughing + deep breathing independently - Turns with minimal assistance - breath sounds clear bilaterally. Abdominal dsg changed - no evidence of redness, swelling noted Janet M. York RN

Figure 7–7 □ Modified source-oriented note. (Courtesy of Hamilton Hospital, Trenton, NJ.)

MERCER MEDICAL CENTER

DIABETES TEACHING GUIDE

Name: _____ Doctor: _____

Age: _____ Room No. _____ History # _____

Address: _____

Home Telephone Number: _____

CONTENT AREAS

PATIENT HAS RECEIVED INSTRUCTION IN THE FOLLOWING:

	*DISCUSSION	FILM	LITERATURE	SIGNATURE
1. Disease Description				
2. Diet				
3. Medications: Oral Hypoglycemics Insulin: Action, peak times, administration.				
4. Urine Testing				
5. Hyperglyemia				
6. Hypoglycemia Insulin Reactions				
7. Foot Care				
8. General Health Practices				
9. Long Term Complications				
10. Blood Glucose Testing				

*Date and sign box under "Discussion" when area has been completed.

FAMILY INSTRUCTION: | COMMENTS:

Figure 7–8 □ Teaching record. (Courtesy of Mercer Medical Center, Trenton, NJ.)

Illustration continued on following page

MANAGEMENT SKILLS

PATIENT IS ABLE TO: PATIENT'S FAMILY IS ABLE TO:

	DATE	SIGNATURE
1. Test and record results for urine sugar and ketones.		
2. Measure and inject insulin using the proper technique.		
3. Recognize the signs and symptoms of an elevated blood sugar and know appropriate action to take.		
4. Recognize the signs and symptoms of low blood sugar reaction and know how to treat accordingly.		
5. Explain the use of oral hypoglycemic agents.		
6. Plan a menu for a few days using the exchange system.		
7. Explain the need for good preventative health measures.		
8. Demonstrate the use of Blood Glucose Monitoring Equipment.		

REFERRALS: COMMENTS:

Developed by: Roseanne Ottaggio, R.N., B.S.N.
               Patient Education Coordinator
               Mercer Medical Center

Figure 7–8 □ *Continued*

fore, data are more accessible and focus on the client's individual needs. The advantages of a problem-oriented system are as follows.

☐ Quality care is facilitated, since the entire health care team focuses on the same identified problems.
☐ All disciplines involved in the care of the client have rapid access to data reflecting the plan of care.
☐ The collaboration of all health team members is encouraged, since multidisciplinary findings are readily available.
☐ Learning is increased because each discipline identifies and observes what others have done.
☐ Evaluation of the quality of care is easily performed and deficiencies more clearly identified.
☐ Research is facilitated, since records tend to be more accurate and complete.

The disadvantages of a problem-oriented system are few but may include the following.

☐ The education of a variety of disciplines in the utilization of the system may be lengthy and costly.
☐ Members of some disciplines may resist the utilization of an integrated system.
☐ Practitioners may have concerns regarding criticism by other disciplines.
☐ If care is fragmented and nonindividualized, documentation will not resolve these problems.

There are four major components of a problem-oriented system: (1) the data base, (2) the problem list, (3) a plan, and (4) the progress notes.

Data Base

The standard data base in a problem-oriented system includes the client's profile, history, and physical and diagnostic studies (e.g., laboratory and radiology reports). The nurse's involvement in the collection of the data base is frequently dependent upon the practice setting. Nurses in hospitals may complete a portion of this record if integrated, or they may utilize an adapted form that reflects the areas of nursing responsibility. Nurses in other settings, such as community health, collaborative practice, or mental health centers, may be responsible for acquiring all components of the data base. The information acquired becomes the source from which the client's needs and problems are identified. The methods for acquiring an accurate and complete data base have been discussed in detail in Chapter 2.

Problem List

The problem list is a cumulative listing of actual or potential client problems that may require intervention to improve the client's health or well-being. Problems may be identified independently by specific health care providers or collaboratively in client care conferences. The problem list is usually on the front of the chart and serves as the index or table of contents to the medical record. It includes the diagnoses of nursing, medicine, and other disciplines. Each problem on the list is designated by number (Table 7–2). This number reflects the sequence in which the problems have been identified, rather than their priority or intensity.

Although the number remains fixed, the status of each problem is dynamic. It may be active, in the process of resolution, or inactive. Signs or symptoms may appear as components of the problem list to indicate the need for further investigation. If the client's condition improves and the sign or symptom subsides, it is eliminated from the problem list. If it persists, a diagnostic label is formulated, and it becomes an active component of the problem list. When a problem is resolved, the date is entered; however, the number assigned to the problem is not used to identify subsequent problems.

In Table 7–2, problems 1 and 2 have been resolved, while 3, 4, and 5 are active. Problems 4a and b are symptoms that may be resolved through treatment of 3 or 4 or may then become additions to the problem list.

Plan

After identifying a problem, the health care provider must develop a plan of care for the client. Initial plans usually include diagnostic, therapeutic, and educational components. The diagnostic component includes the acquisition of additional data required to confirm the diagnosis (whether medical, nursing, or other). This may consist of laboratory or radiology studies, such as urinalysis or chest x-ray. It may also include gathering

TABLE 7–2 □ **PROBLEM LIST**

No.	Problem	Date Entered	Date Resolved
1	Cholecystitis	1963	1963
2	Pneumonia	1972	1972
3	Fractured left hip	2/2/86	
4	Impaired physical mobility	2/2/86	
	a. Pain	2/3/86	
	b. Edema	2/3/86	
5	Potential for injury	2/4/86	

TABLE 7-3 □ CARE PLAN FOR A PROBLEM FROM TABLE 7-2

Problem 5	Outcome	Orders
Potential for injury	No evidence of further accident or injury	□ Consultation with ophthalmologist to evaluate visual acuity (diagnostic) □ Assist client to identify potential environmental hazards in the home (treatment) □ Instruct client and son in basic safety measures designed to prevent injury (education)

additional data from the client—e.g., from available support systems or the client's feelings—or observation of specific skills or limitations.

Treatment might include intravenous therapy, frequent position change, range of motion exercises, and so on. Education involves providing the client or family with the information and skills required to manage the client's illness or limitations. Table 7-3 reflects a sample plan for problem 5 on the problem list in Table 7-2. Note that outcomes are defined and specific orders necessary to achieve them are included.

Progress Notes

The final component of the problem-oriented system is the progress notes. These are designed to document the client's response to the plan. Integrated progress notes include narrative entries from all disciplines. Evaluation of the information documented in these notes assists in measuring the client's progress toward outcome attainment. This also allows the evaluator to modify the plan accordingly. The freqency of the recording of progress notes may vary depending upon the setting or specific institutional policies. They may be done hourly, once each shift, daily, monthly, or only when significant changes occur.

The format for progress notes in this system is specific and structured. This format is identified by the acronym SOAPE, in which the letters represent Subjective data, Objective data, Assessment, Plan, and Evaluation. Subjective data include the client's feelings, symptoms, and concerns—e.g., fears about the outcome of diagnostic studies. Objective data include the findings of various members of the health team—e.g., lung sounds, blood pressure, or radiology reports. Assessment includes the nurse's interpretation of the subjective and objective data. The plan is the steps that will be taken to assist the client with the resolution of the problem. The evaluation is based on the client's responses to the interventions.

TABLE 7–4 □ **SOAPE PROGRESS NOTES**

Date/Time	Problem	Notes
12/27/85 8:30 A.M.	4	S—"I'm going to have to watch myself when I go home—I don't want to hurt myself again." O—Tense, wringing hands, expresses concern about hurting self. A—Aware of the relationship between hazards in the home and occurrence of injuries. Motivated to avoid harm to self. P—Encourage to reorganize and correct hazards in home environment. E—Plans to request home hazard survey by visiting nurse prior to discharge.

Table 7–4 is a sample of progress notes utilizing the SOAPE format. Note that the problem continues to be identified by number.

It is not necessary to include each component of the format in every set of progress notes. For example, there may be no subjective data if the client is unable to communicate. Therefore, no entries would be included in the S area.

Computer-Assisted Records

The expansion of computerized information systems in health care agencies has resulted in the development of a variety of documentation methods. Some systems generate a shift worksheet similar to the one shown in Figure 7–9. The seven sections define the independent and dependent nursing activities for each client on a given shift. The worksheet reflects the nursing care plan and includes those client outcomes and nursing interventions that are appropriate for each shift. The nurse initials the actions that have been implemented. The nurses' notes are handwritten in a format similar to a source-oriented documentation system. Physicians' orders and nursing interventions may be handwritten on the worksheet after they are entered into the system. Discontinued orders may be deleted from the system at any time. After removing the orders from the computer, the nurse draws a line through the order on the worksheet. This process ensures that orders are current and that documentation reflects the actual care delivered (Hinson et al, 1984).

Other computerized systems utilize a problem-oriented type of documentation. The data base is initiated at the bedside, and a problem list

```
                    P A T I E N T   C A R E   P R O F I L E
      GENERAL HOSPITAL        5/16/84   11:45AM           PAGE  1        SHIFT:1
```

ACTIVITIES OF DAILY LIVING	TRN-09 000187023 2555555 TRN

ACTIVITIES OF DAILY LIVING
  Vital Signs   RT
  OOB   W/Assist
  Bath   W/Assist
  Fluids   Force
  Transport by W/C
All   Regular
Cranberry Juice at Bedside
NPO After Midnight
PRC: Hard of Hearing

—————————————————————

ACTIVE ORDERS
CBC W DIFF   05/16 07:30A
SMA 18 BIOCHEM PRO   05/16 07:30A
PYELOGRAM INTRAVEN   05/16 AM
1: MAY HAVE LIQUIDS ON THE DAY OF EXAM
   UNLESS UPPER G.I.SERIES,GALL
   BLADDER SERIES OR SONOGRAM IS
   ORDERED

—————————————————————

TREATMENTS
1: ANESTHESIA TO SEE PT.
2: SHAVE AND PREP-MID NIPPLE TO MID
   BACK AND FROM MID AXILLA TO HIP ON
   RIGHT SIDE
3: PRE OP ON CALL.   DATE:5/17
4: STRAIN ALL URINE. D/E/N:
5: INTAKE & OUTPUT q SHIFT.
   D/E/N:

TRN-09   000187023 2555555   TRN
TESTPAT JACK   SEX: M
ADM: 5/15/84   SRV: URO   SMK: N
DOB: 10/06/21   62 COND: G LEVEL: 1
HT: 5/11 F/I   WT: 180/000 P/O
10000 INTERNIST OTHER
ALG: PENICILLIN
DX: NEPHROLITHIASIS

—————————————————————

OUTCOME: Describes type of surgery
OUTCOME: States usual pre-op
         preparation
OUTCOME: Identifies usual post-op
         routine
OUTCOME: Verbalizes feelings about
         impending surgery
INTERVENTIONS:
1: Assess knowledge of surgery and
   explore past surgical experience(s)
   at the time of admission
2: Review surgical routine (preps,
   meds, dressing)
3: Reinforce pre-operative teaching
   re: Sequence of events on day of
   surgery (pre-op stretcher to
   O.R., R.R. return to room/ICU)
   Post-op equipment (dsg., I.V.,
   tubes)
   Provisions for relief of pain
   and other symptoms (include
   need to request and frequency
   limitations)
   Turning, coughing and deep
   breathing
   Incentive spirometry if ordered
   Change in bowel/bladder
   functions
   Progressive diet changes
   Progressive self care

—————————————————————

DATE: NURSING NOTES   SIGNATURE

[Handwritten nursing notes:]

8am Clear yellow urine. No evidence of stones or (R) flank pain.
Pt. prepared for IVP this am. Dr. Jones visited — Pat Kelly, Rn
10³⁰ am Returned from X-ray. Demerol 100mg. IM RUO for
(R) flank pain — Sally Smith, Rn
11⁸ pm Pain subsided. Pt. verbalized understanding of
information in pre-op booklet and able to give return
demonstration of TCDB. — Pat Kelly, Rn
1³⁰ pm Urine remains clear. No evidence of stones or (R) flank pain.
— Pat Kelly, Rn

INT	SIGNATURE	INT	SIGNATURE	INT	SIGNATURE
PK	Pat Kelly, Rn	SS	Sally Smith, Rn		

Figure 7–9 □ Computer-generated shift worksheet. (Courtesy of HBO & Company, Atlanta, GA. All rights reserved.)

is generated. The computer identifies unusual or abnormal findings and prioritizes those areas requiring additional attention. Each problem is addressed in the initial plan in order of priority. The nurse selects diagnoses, sets client outcomes, and chooses nursing orders. (If standardized care plans are available in the system, this process may be expedited.)

Progress notes may be documented by using one of two approaches. The nurse may choose specific interventions to document. "The computer presents any appropriate descriptions associated with the order for elaboration" (McNeill, 1980). These may be simple statements (such as "completed" or "not completed") or more detailed descriptions of care. The system then sorts the information provided into subjective and objective data and follows the SOAPE format. The second approach builds the progress notes by selection of data from displays. This allows documentation of current data and the addition of new findings. The nurse chooses from structured screens in the SOAPE format. These screens contain significant symptoms and physical findings that serve as a guideline for additional assessment and nursing management. The progress notes of all disciplines are documented in an integrated fashion.

A number of additional forms may be used to document nursing interventions, such as administration of medications. The form is generated by the computer, and the nurse initials those medications administered to the client.

SUMMARY

Implementation is the phase of the nursing process that involves the initiation of the nursing care plan. The goal of implementation is the achievement of outcomes. The implementation phase is divided into three stages—preparation, interventions, and documentation. Preparation includes reviewing anticipated nursing actions, analyzing the nursing knowledge and skills required, and recognizing the potential complications associated with specific nursing orders. Preparation also involves determining and providing necessary resources, preparing an environment conducive to the types of interventions required, and identifying the ethical and legal concerns associated with potential interventions.

The client's physical and emotional needs may be divided into 11 functional health patterns. While each has an infinite variety of interventions associated with it, assessment, planning, and teaching are common approaches.

Documentation, the last stage, may utilize source-oriented, problem-oriented, or computer-assisted records.

7–1   TEST YOURSELF

DOCUMENTATION OF IMPLEMENTATION

Charles Stewart is a 67 year old man who was admitted to the hospital two days ago with a diagnosis of anorexia. The following is a segment of his care plan.

Nursing Diagnosis	Outcomes	Nursing Plan
Alteration in nutrition (less than body requirements) related to anorexia	No evidence of significant weight change	1. Provide small frequent meals at 8 A.M., 1 P.M., 4 P.M., 6 P.M. 2. Supplemental feeding: Ensure 90 ml at 11 A.M. and 9 P.M. 3. Assess likes/dislikes. 4. Encourage food from home if permitted. 5. Obtain dietary consult (date: 7/5) 6. Monitor food intake. 7. Weigh daily at 8 A.M.

While you are caring for Mr. Stewart, he shares the following information with you. "I don't like strawberry Ensure, although the other flavors are all right. What I'd really like would be some of my wife's lasagna or bread pudding." When Mr. Stewart's trays were observed after each meal, you noted that he consumed all of his breakfast, two thirds of his lunch, and 45 ml of Ensure at 11 A.M. His weight at 8 A.M. was 148 lb, which constitutes a loss of three pounds since admission. Therefore you suggest to Mr. Stewart's physician that a consultation with a dietician be obtained. She agrees, and the dietician visits at 1:30 P.M.

Based on the information provided above, document the implementation of this segment of the plan of care using source-oriented, modified source oriented, or SOAPE format.

7-1 TEST YOURSELF □ ANSWERS

Source-Oriented

Date	Time	Nurses' Notes
7/5/85	8 A.M.	Discussed dietary preferences with client—indicates that he wants "my wife's lasagna or bread pudding." Weight 148 lb this A.M. Consumed entire breakfast.
	10:00	Dr. Klein visited—discussed weight loss—dietary consult order requested and received.
	11:00	Consumed ½ Ensure feeding. Client indicates that he "hates the strawberry Ensure although the other flavors are all right."
	1 P.M.	Consumed ⅔ of lunch.
	1:30	Visited by K. Moore, R.D.—will make changes in diet and discontinue strawberry Ensure.
	2:00	Wife visited—encouraged to bring in foods from home.
		Janet York, R.N.

Modified Source-Oriented

Date/Time	Diagnosis	Nurses' Notes
7/5/85 3 P.M.	Nutrition	Dietary preferences reviewed with client at 8 A.M.—indicates that he wants "my wife's lasagna or bread pudding." Weight at this time 148 lb. Consumed all of breakfast, ⅔ lunch, and ½ of 11 A.M. Ensure feeding. Indicates that he "hates the strawberry Ensure although the other flavors are all right." Dr. Klein visited at 10 A.M.—weight loss discussed. Dietary consult order requested and received. K. Moore, R.D., visited at 1:30 P.M.—will make changes in diet and discontinue strawberry Ensure. Wife visited at 2:30 P.M.—encouraged to bring in food from home.
		Janet York, R.N.

SOAPE Note

Date	Time	
7/5/85	8 A.M.	S: "I don't like strawberry Ensure. I'd like some of my wife's lasagna or bread pudding."

	O: Weight 148 lb. Consumed all of his breakfast.
11 A.M.	Drank 45 ml of Ensure.
12 P.M.	Ate ⅔ of his lunch.
	A: Significant weight loss of three pounds since admission probably related to decreased caloric consumption.
12:30 P.M.	*P:* Requested and received order for dietary consult.
1:30 P.M.	*E:* Visited by dietician who will be making changes in diet, and discontinue sending strawberry Ensure.
2 P.M.	Mrs. Stewart willing to bring in favorite foods from home.
	Janet York, R.N.

References

American Hospital Association: A Patient's Bill of Rights. Chicago: American Hospital Association, 1975.

American Nurses' Association: Code for Nurses with Interpretive Statements. Kansas City: American Nurses' Association, 1976.

Carpenito LJ: Nursing Diagnosis—Application to Clinical Practice. Philadelphia: JB Lippincott, 1983.

Cazalas M: Nursing and the Law. Germantown, Md: Aspen, 1978.

Churchill L: Ethical issues of a profession in transition. American Journal of Nursing 873, 1977.

Gordon M: Nursing Diagnosis: Process and Application. New York: McGraw-Hill, 1982.

Hemelt M and Mackert M: Dynamics of Law in Nursing and Health Care. 2nd ed. Reston, Va: Prentice-Hall, 1982.

Hinson I, Nettie S, Clapp P, et al: An automated Kardex and care plan. Nursing Management 35–43, July 1984.

Kelly L: Dimensions of Professional Nursing. 4th ed. New York: Macmillan, 1981.

McNeill D: Developing the complete computer-based information system. In Zielstorff R: Computers in Nursing. Rockville, Md: Aspen, 1982.

Murray M: Fundamentals of Nursing. 2nd ed. Englewood Cliffs, NJ: Prentice-Hall, 1980.

Sorensen K and Luckmann J: Basic Nursing: A Psychophysiologic Approach. Philadelphia: WB Saunders, 1979.

Bibliography

Aiken L: Nursing in the '80's: Crises, Opportunities, Challenges. Philadelphia: JB Lippincott, 1982.

Cross J and Thomas G: Plans, implementation and scientific rationale. In Griffith K and Christensen P: Nursing Process. St. Louis: CV Mosby, 1982.

Eggland E: Charting: How and why to document your care daily and fully. Nursing 38–43, February 1980.

Ellis J and Hartley C: Nursing in Today's World. 2nd ed. Philadelphia: JB Lippincott, 1984.

Kerr A: Nurses' notes—that's where the goodies are! Nursing 34–41, February 1975.

Kozier B and Erb G: Fundamentals of Nursing Concepts and Procedures. Menlo Park, Calif: Addison-Wesley, 1979.

LaMonica E: Nursing Process. Menlo Park, Calif: Addison-Wesley, 1979.

Marriner M: A Systematic Approach to the Nursing Care Plan. Norwalk, Conn: Appleton-Century-Crofts, 1983.
Mitchell P: Concepts Basic to Nursing. 2nd ed. New York: McGraw-Hill, 1977.
Rutkowski B: How DRG's are changing your charting. Nursing 49–51, October 1985.
Zielstorff R (ed): Computers in Nursing. Rockville, Md: Aspen, 1982.

8

Implementation— Nursing Care Delivery Systems

Regardless of the type of setting in which nurses practice, usually one of three major models is utilized for implementing nursing care. These three approaches are (1) functional nursing, (2) team nursing, and (3) primary nursing. Their differences lie primarily in the systems used by nurses to organize and carry out the types of activities necessary to satisfy client needs. Nursing care may be accomplished by using individual models in their pure form or by adapting one or more methods. The following will explore each of the three models in terms of its definition, advantages, and disadvantages.

FUNCTIONAL NURSING

Definition

In the functional approach to nursing care delivery, nursing responsibilities are divided by task and performed by varying levels of nursing personnel. All caregivers are involved in the client's care, but each individual is assigned to complete selected functions, such as monitoring vital signs, administering medications, or giving treatments. The individual functions are assigned to various levels of personnel based on the complexity

225

of the task, including the knowledge, skills, and experience required to complete them.

For example, on an individual nursing unit on any given day, one RN may be in charge of unit management, another administers medications, and a third completes patient teaching. The LPN may be assigned to measure vital signs or bathe clients, while the nursing assistant makes beds or delivers meal trays.

In an office setting, the LPNs may take patient histories, record vital signs, and perform simple treatments. The RN similarly accomplishes physical assessment, administers medications, completes complex treatments, and provides education to the client.

Advantages

1. The emphasis in this model is on the efficient delivery of required care. Since the system allows the use of less skilled personnel to complete many tasks, it may also be more economical. Individual staff members become more skilled and efficient when assigned to the same tasks on a regular basis. This may also more effectively utilize the individual nurse's skills and experience. Some nurses are particularly skilled at initiating intravenous therapy or administering medications and tend to be more motivated and efficient when completing those tasks than when performing treatments or teaching clients.

2. The volume of supplies and equipment required may also be decreased because fewer numbers of personnel utilize them. Consistency of task assignment may also decrease maintenance costs of equipment, since staff members become more proficient in the use of the types of equipment required to complete their specific function.

3. This method also tends to facilitate the organization of work, since assignments are clearly defined. Therefore, the overlapping of responsibilities and the associated confusion are minimized.

Disadvantages

1. The primary concern with the functional model is the fragmentation of care to which it gives rise. Assigning a variety of personnel to specific tasks frequently becomes inefficient and impersonal. The client is often divided into segments, each of which must be managed by a different individual. One nurse takes care of medications, a second

undertakes teaching, and a third monitors vital signs. This tends to make the client feel insecure and frustrated.

2. Continuity of care is difficult, if not impossible, since no single staff member has a complete picture of the client's needs and responses to nursing or medical interventions. This allows unnoticed gaps to occur in client care.

3. From the nurse's perspective, this type of care delivery may become monotonous. Administration of medications for weeks at a time may decrease the nurse's motivation and limits continued personal development because of reduced exposure to a variety of experiences.

4. Job satisfaction may also be diminished in a functional approach because the individual nurse's role in the client's recovery may not be clearly defined or perceived as valuable by the client, other staff members, or supervisory personnel.

5. Communication and decision-making may be compromised, since caregivers are focusing on individual aspects of the client's care. Frequently, the nurse manager is the only staff member who receives complete information on the client. The responsibility and accountability for decision-making is focused on the manager rather than individual staff members who actually implement the plan of care.

TEAM NURSING

Definition

Team nursing is a system of nursing care delivery in which a group of professional and nonprofessional personnel work together to deliver nursing care to a number of clients. It was designed after World War II (1) to provide improved client care utilizing available staff and (2) to alleviate the problems associated with the functional method (Tappen, 1983). Team nursing is frequently utilized in nursing homes, hospitals, and community health settings. Comprehensive client care is provided by the staff member under the direction of a registered nurse who is the team leader. Other team members may include RNs, LPNs, and nursing assistants. However, the size and composition of a team are often dependent upon the setting.

The team leader is the key person in this model. Leaders must have particular knowledge and skills not only in client care procedures and techniques but also in management and decision-making strategies. The team leader has the authority and responsibility for assigning the care of a group of clients to team members. These assignments are based on client needs and the knowledge, skills, and experiences of team members.

The success of the team approach is dependent upon effective communication. This method relies on the use of written client care assignments, timely development and revision of nursing care plans, frequent participation in client care conferences, and frequent reports and feedback among team members.

Advantages

1. Although nursing care in a team approach is divided among several staff members, it is less fragmented than in the functional method. This is a result of the extensive communication and coordination built into the system. Continuity of care is facilitated, particularly in systems where teams are constant. Therefore, team nursing is more satisfying to clients, since they are able to identify and communicate more effectively with the personnel responsible for delivering care.

2. From the nurse's perspective, the team model is more satisfying because the skills of each team member are frequently identified, recognized, and utilized. This provides the opportunity for nurses to identify their role in the client's progress along the illness-wellness continuum. The participation of team members in client care conferences improves the quality of decision-making and facilitates the development of individual team members. The cooperation and communication inherent in the system increase the potential for the delivery of quality nursing care.

Disadvantages

1. The team nursing model can very easily become a duplication of the functional method. For example, if team members are responsible for individual functions, such as administering medications, monitoring vital signs, or giving baths, it is difficult to differentiate this system from functional team nursing.

2. Team nursing may be less efficient than a functional system. The communication and coordination required for the success of the system are compromised if the team leader does not have skills in organization, leadership, communication, motivation, and nursing care delivery. This method can also be ineffective if staff members are not client-centered, skilled in nursing practice, and able to communicate clearly.

3. The number of personnel caring for clients is not substantially

reduced in a team approach. This may not be cost-effective and may dilute the quality of care provided, particularly in settings in which a large volume of nonnursing personnel provide direct care.

4. The dilution of individual responsibility and accountability may also decrease the quality of care provided.

PRIMARY NURSING

Definition

Primary nursing is a system of care delivery in which the registered nurse is responsible and accountable for directing the care of a client. The primary nurse develops the plan of care and ensures that the plan is implemented around the clock. In the absence of the primary nurse, the care of the client is delegated to an associate nurse, who follows the plan of care as developed by the primary nurse.

Primary nursing may be utilized in a variety of settings, including hospitals and public health agencies. Primary nursing systems emphasize (1) the nurse's responsibility and accountability for management of care, (2) the importance of accurate and complete assessment, diagnosis, and planning, (3) the client's involvement in validation and goal-setting, (4) the need for communication between primary nurses and other nurses, members of the health care team, and clients and their families, and (5) preparation for discharge through client and family teaching, identification of available resources, and referral to other systems when required.

In some settings, primary nurses select their own clients. More frequently, the unit is divided into districts or modules, with one primary nurse assigned to each area. This nurse provides direct care to a caseload, which usually does not exceed six clients. The head nurse functions as the coordinator of the unit and is a resource person for the primary nurses. The primary nurse plans and provides the care, administers medications and treatments, interacts with the physician and other health professionals, and reports on the client's status. Other levels of staff, including LPNs and nursing assistants, aid the primary nurse in the provision of care. Client care conferences, which involve primary and associate nurses as well as other members of the health team, are frequently utilized to discuss specific client problems and to develop strategies for resolving them.

The professional nurse functioning in a primary care setting must have (1) a thorough knowledge of the nursing process, (2) refined communication skills, (3) the ability to perform nursing procedures identified in nursing orders, (4) well-developed problem-solving techniques, and (5) a commitment to client-centered care.

Advantages

1. The primary nursing method of delivery promotes consistent, total client care by virtue of the quality and frequency of interactions between the client and the nurse. Each primary nurse is responsible for coordinating all aspects of care, including physical and emotional care, teaching, and the medical regimen.

2. This method promotes increased autonomy and responsibility in individual nursing practice. The nurse may be more satisfied because involvement in direct care is increased, and therefore the nurse's role in the client's recovery is more clearly defined. Additionally, the nurse is more accountable, since care responsibilities focus on the total care of a small number of clients rather than the partial care of many.

3. Primary nursing also provides the opportunity for professional growth. The nurse's involvement in all aspects of the client's care, particularly the decision-making component, facilitates the acquisition of new knowledge and skills. Nurses frequently feel that they are more effective in a primary system because they have a more global view of the needs of the client and family.

4. Clients are also generally more satisfied because of the increased frequency of interaction with one specific nurse who is particularly knowledgeable about them. This allows the client to identify clearly the primary nurse and creates an atmosphere of trust and open communication.

5. Other health care providers, such as physicians, therapists, and dieticians, also appreciate the ability to interact with an individual nurse who is informed about the client.

Disadvantages

1. Primary nursing requires competent practitioners who can function independently when implementing the nursing process. Not all nurses are comfortable in accepting the responsibility associated with this system.

2. In some instances, primary nursing may be less economical than functional or team nursing, since this model may require a larger percentage of registered nurses.

Table 8–1 summarizes functional, team, and primary nursing.

Text continued on page 236

TABLE 8–1 □ NURSING CARE DELIVERY SYSTEMS

Factor	Functional	Team	Primary
Assignments	Head nurse or nursing coordinator assigns to staff members tasks that fall within their job descriptions.	Team leader assigns to team members tasks that fall within their job descriptions.	Head nurse or nursing coordinator assigns individual clients to professional nurses, matching the client's need to the nurse's skills.
Assessment, planning, and evaluation	Related to specific needs of each client; done by any member of the nursing staff; no continuity.	Related to specific needs of each client; done by the team leader; limited continuity, depending on how long a person remains team leader.	Related to specific needs of each client; done by the primary nurse; maximum continuity, since primary nurse remains throughout client's stay on hospital unit.
Implementation	Different members of the nursing staff do tasks for a given client.	Each team member does tasks for all clients according to job description; the team leader often does medications and charting for the team.	Each primary nurse delivers total care to all assigned clients. ("For the first time I feel that somebody knows who I am.")
Documentation	Staff members make notations on only those actions or aspects of care done by them. *Or* a staff member is assigned to "chart" for a given number of clients. Usually no nursing care plan is in evidence.	Team leader usually documents care of clients cared for by most, or all, team members; sometimes a team member makes some entries on client charts; the team leader documents the nursing care plan.	Each primary or associate nurse documents care given to each assigned client during shift; the primary nurse documents the nursing care plan.

Table continued on following page

TABLE 8-1 □ NURSING CARE DELIVERY SYSTEMS *Continued*

Factor	Functional	Team	Primary
Reporting at end of shift	A "charge" nurse reports on patients to another charge nurse; most of the information shared is based on reports of other workers.	The team leader gives report on the group of clients to the oncoming team; most of the information shared is based on reports of other workers.	The primary nurse gives a report on each assigned client to oncoming nurse who will care for the client; the nurse who reports has interacted directly with all the clients about whom reports are given.
Responsibility for planning care	No one person is responsible for planning unless this is assigned as a functional task to a specific RN for a given period.	The team leader is responsible for planning the nursing care for the assigned group of clients.	The primary nurse is responsible for planning the nursing care of all primary clients, from the time they are admitted to a nursing unit until they are discharged from that unit.
Responsibility for providing care	Nursing care is delivered in a fragmented manner—many staff members interact with the client as the various tasks are done.	As in functional nursing, delivery of nursing care is a "mixed bag."	The primary nurse directly delivers all nursing care to the primary clients when on duty.
Decentralization of authority, for continuous decision-making and follow-up on nursing care	Total decentralization—decisions are made on basis of separate tasks done by individual staff members for each client on the unit.	The team leader makes final decisions about nursing care for the clients in the group on basis of feedback (some of which is lost) from team members.	Each primary nurse makes final decisions about nursing care for the assigned clients.
Accountability (to clients, families, peers, physicians, interdepartmental staff, administration, community)			

For professional actions	Professional nurses are answerable for their own professional actions.	Professional nurses are answerable for their own professional actions.	Professional nurses are answerable for their own professional actions.
For coordination and outcomes of nursing care	No one nursing staff member is answerable for the coordination and outcomes of nursing care; the head nurse often answers to everyone for the entire staff.	The team leader, who plans care but often does not give it, is answerable for the care of each client in the assigned group and for the coordination and outcomes of nursing care.	The primary nurse who plans and delivers the care to each assigned client is answerable for the coordination and outcomes of nursing care.
For follow-up on client problems	Physicians, administrators, and other interdepartmental personnel can rarely pinpoint responsibility for follow-up on problems.	The team leader is responsible for follow-up on client problems, which are often generated by other staff.	The primary nurse is responsible for follow-up on problems of assigned clients.
—"Passing the buck?"	"Passing the buck" prevalent.	Moderate amount of "buck-passing" because of change in staff assignments from day to day.	Minimal, if any, "passing the buck" because of constancy of staff assignments to same clients.
Comprehensiveness of care, in terms of Clients' needs	Not possible; focus of care is on tasks, not on the client as a unique individual with a broad spectrum of needs and resources.	Theoretically and sometimes actually possible, since team members are expected to communicate ideas related to client needs and nursing actions to meet those needs; a united approach is the goal; however, plans are often designed with minimal client or family input, and focus is on nursing actions rather than on client outcomes.	Inherent in the system because continuity in same nurse/same client relationships is maximized; focus of nursing care is on client outcomes rather than on nursing actions.

Table continued on following page

TABLE 8–1 □ NURSING CARE DELIVERY SYSTEMS *Continued*

Factor	Functional	Team	Primary
Documentation	Nursing care regimens are rarely documented, so individual approaches are inconsistent.	Documented nursing care plans are encouraged but can rarely be demanded because nursing case load is too large.	Documented nursing care plans are mandated by smaller case load of each nurse and by constancy of assignment.
Communication Between nurses and clients	Client, family, and significant others find it difficult to identify a nursing staff member with whom to relate on a continuing basis.	Client, family, and significant others may be confused as to identity of the nursing staff member to whom questions and problems may be directed.	Client, family, and significant others can clearly identify the nurse and can share ideas, feelings, and problems freely with this person.
Between nurses and staff of other departments	Physicians, administrators, and interdepartmental staff address questions and problems to nurses or to head nurse on unit, but often satisfactory answers are delayed or are not available.	Same as in functional nursing, except team leader rather than head nurse may be consulted.	All communications are directed to the primary nurse for each client. Satisfactory answers are more likely to be forthcoming. Persons may find difficulty in locating specific nurses.
Between nurses and supervisors	Instructions often have to be repeated because of changes in staff assignments and lack of consistent documentation of nursing care plans.	Same as in functional nursing.	Dramatic decrease in repetition of instructions for particular client due to constancy of assignments and mandatory care plans.

Cost-effectiveness	Not cost-effective because	Not cost-effective because	Most likely to be cost-effective because
	1. Product (nursing care) is of poor quality owing to fragmentation; this results in many complaints from clients.	1. Product is of only moderate quality, since expertise in judgment and communication cannot be delegated from the care-planners (team leaders) to the caregivers (team members).	1. Product is of high quality since the person most prepared and best equipped to perform does so on a continuing basis for the same clients.
	2. Nursing staff easily becomes frustrated, and turnover rate is usually high, thus increasing cost of orientation and of staff development.	2. Turnover of nursing staff is moderate but variable.	2. Turnover of nursing staff is minimal because of higher level of satisfaction experienced by nurses.
	3. Output from professional nurses is low since they are not required to perform the full job—the total nursing process—for which they are being paid.	3. Same as for functional nursing.	3. Professional nurses do the job for which they are being paid; "unproductive" time decreases dramatically.

Adapted from Kron T: Management of Patient Care. 5th ed. Philadelphia: WB Saunders, 1981.

SUMMARY

Functional, team, and primary nursing are three methods of delivering nursing care. The differences among the systems are dependent upon the mechanisms utilized by nurses to organize and deliver care. Each method has advantages that influence the efficiency and effectiveness of the system.

Reference

Tappen R: Nursing Leadership: Concept and Practice. Philadelphia: FA Davis, 1983.

Bibliography

Aiken L: Nursing in the 80's: Crises, Opportunities, Challenges. Philadelphia: JB Lippincott, 1982.
Chavigny K and Lewis A: Team or primary nursing care? Nursing Outlook 322–27, November/December 1984.
Kelley L: Dimensions of Professional Nursing. 4th ed. New York: Macmillan, 1981.
Kron T: The Management of Patient Care. 5th ed. Philadelphia: WB Saunders, 1981.
LaMonica F: Nursing Process. Menlo Park, Calif: Addison-Wesley, 1979.
Mackay C and Ault L: A systematic approach to individualized nursing care. Journal of Nursing Administration 39–48, January, 1977.
Marriner A: Nursing Process. St. Louis: CV Mosby, 1979.

9

Evaluation

Evaluation is defined as the planned, systematic comparison of the client's health status with the outcomes. By measuring the client's progress toward meeting the objectives, the nurse judges the effectiveness of nursing actions (Griffith and Christensen, 1982).

EVALUATION OF GOAL ACHIEVEMENT

The evaluation process consists of two steps:
1. Gathering data about the client's health status;
2. Comparing gathered data with the outcomes and making a judgment about the client's progress toward achievement of outcomes.

Gathering Data

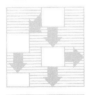

The nurse uses assessment skills to gather data for the purposes of evaluation. Several aspects of the client's health status are evaluated. These include the areas for which outcomes are written:
1. Appearance and functioning of the body;
2. Specific symptoms;

237

3. Knowledge;
4. Psychomotor skills;
5. Emotional status.

Appearance and Functioning of the Body

The outcomes written for this component cover a number of readily observable aspects of the client's health status. To evaluate outcome attainment, the nurse focuses on how the appearance and functioning of the body have changed as a result of nursing interventions. Either direct observation of the client or examination of the chart may be used to gather data for purposes of evaluation.

Direct Observation. Direct observation should involve careful and thorough assessment of the client's appearance and activities. These data are compared with prior baseline data that were gathered at some previous point in time. Baseline data may have been gathered during the initial assessment of the client or during subsequent interactions. The new data are compared with the client's previous condition and used to judge the effectiveness of nursing interventions.

Example. *Outcome:* Throughout hospitalization, no evidence of skin breakdown over bony prominences. To evaluate this outcome, the nurse would carefully inspect the client's skin, paying particular attention to the sacrum, elbows, hips, and heels. The inspection would occur as an ongoing part of care while the client was being bathed or positioned. These findings would be compared with initial baseline data or subsequent observations.

Examination of the Chart. Review of the client's medical record is useful in evaluating the functions of the client's body. The nurse notes how the client's condition has changed as a result of nursing care. The results of studies, such as blood gases, blood glucose, chest x-rays, electrolytes, or urinalysis, may be useful in evaluating the client's progress. To gain a complete picture of the status of the client, the nurse also notes the response to the treatments of other departments, such as respiratory, occupational, or physical therapy.

Example. *Outcome:* Has balanced intake and output within 48 hours. To evaluate this outcome, the nurse would analyze the intake and output and look for any discrepancies between the two. If differences are found, the nurse would identify the causes and take appropriate action, such as increasing intake or notifying the physician.

Specific Symptoms

Outcomes are written to measure the reduction or alleviation of symptoms that are affecting the client's health status. These outcomes can be evaluated through direct observation, client interview, or examination of the chart.

Direct Observation. In some cases, direct observation will yield data about the current status of the client's response to illness.

Example. Outcome: No evidence of wheezing within 48 hours. To evaluate this outcome, the nurse would listen to the client's breath sounds on the anterior and posterior aspects of the chest.

Client Interview. Discussion with the client will provide the nurse with information about the client's symptoms. Symptoms are subjective in nature. Therefore, they are best evaluated by eliciting information from the client.

Example. Outcome: Expresses alleviation of discomfort within one hour following initiation of comfort measure. To evaluate this outcome, the nurse would ask the client whether the pain has subsided since the medication was given.

Examination of the Chart. Other symptoms are best evaluated by looking for a pattern of response, which may be documented in the record and may include those aspects of the client's progress that can be measured in units.

Examples

☐ Weight loss or gain
☐ Temperature elevations
☐ Frequency of a symptom's occurrence, such as pain or vomiting
☐ Duration of symptom (time in minutes, hours, or days)

The nurse can review flowsheets, progress notes, and graphic records to compare the client's current status with baseline data.

Example. Outcome: Temperature within normal limits 48 hours post-op. To evaluate this outcome, the nurse would examine the temperature graph, noting any elevations in temperature.

Knowledge

Outcomes identify the specific knowledge that the client should acquire as a result of teaching. Specific areas to evaluate include the client's knowledge of the disease, symptom control, medications, diet, activities, resources in the community, potential complications, symptoms that should be reported, preventive measures, and so on. Outcomes pertaining to knowledge can be evaluated through the use of client interviews or paper and pencil tests.

Client Interview. Frequently, the best way to evaluate the client's knowledge is through an interview. The nurse may use several strategies to assess the client's level of understanding of what has been taught. These may include

☐ *Recall of knowledge*—ask the client to remember certain facts. "Let's review. Why are you supposed to eat foods high in potassium if you are taking a diuretic?"
☐ *Comprehension of knowledge*—ask the client to state specific information in his or her own words. "Could you tell me how you would know if your blood sugar was low?"
☐ *Application of facts*—present the client with a hypothetical situation and ask what would be an appropriate action. "Suppose you are alone when your baby stops breathing. What would you do?"

Paper and Pencil Tests. Nurses sometimes use paper and pencil tests to evaluate a client's knowledge of material that has been taught. The advantage of such an approach is that the test is an objective tool that will measure the same information each time it is used. There are disadvantages, however: tests are difficult to construct, frequently intimidate the client, and are of little value for clients with low reading skills.

Psychomotor Skills

Psychomotor skills are fairly easy to evaluate if observable behavior has been identified in the outcome. This is usually accomplished by direct observation. Watching the client perform specific activities is the most appropriate way to evaluate psychomotor skills. The nurse compares the actual performance with the behavior described in the outcome. If the client is hospitalized, the equipment used to teach and evaluate psychomotor skills should be identical to the materials the client will be using at home.

Example. Outcome: By the end of the teaching session, injects insulin using correct technique. To evaluate this outcome, the nurse would give the client a syringe and vial of insulin and observe whether the client (1) draws out the correct amount of insulin without contaminating the syringe, (2) selects an appropriate skin site and prepares the surface, (3) inserts the needle at a 90° angle, (4) injects the insulin, and (5) withdraws the needle and massages the site.

Emotional Status

The emotions that the client is experiencing are subjective and tend to be difficult to measure. Therefore, the outcomes are written in terms of the behaviors that will give an indication of the client's emotional status. The outcomes include phrases such as "shares feelings about," "reports less anxiety," "initiates conversations" (if depressed), and so on. This wording enables the nurse to evaluate attainment of the outcomes.

Direct Observation. Interactions with the client are useful in evaluating emotional status. The nurse observes facial expression, body posture, and tone of voice as well as the content of verbal messages.

Feedback from Other Staff. As is true in evaluating any aspect of the client's health status, it is important to gather data from as many sources as possible. The nurse can confer with other personnel to validate observations about the client. There are many opportunities to share information, including informal conversations, patient-centered conferences, and change of shift reports as well as reading observations recorded by other staff in the client's record.

Making Judgments about Progress

After gathering data about the client's health status, the nurse compares the data with the outcome. The next step involves making judgment about the client's achievement of the outcome. There are three possibilities in this regard.

1. The client has achieved the outcome. In this case, the nurse would assess the client for further problems or evaluate attainment of other outcomes.

Example. William Hawk is a 67 year old retired welder who was overweight and physically inactive. With the assistance of the visiting nurse, he was able to achieve the outcome of establishing a regular exercise pattern. Then Mr. Hawk was able to focus on his second goal—to lose 20 pounds in two months. His nurse continued to assist with meal planning until the weight loss was accomplished.

2. The client is in the process of achieving the outcome. The nurse recognizes that the client is moving toward resolution of the problem.

Additional time, resources, and interventions may be needed before the outcome is achieved.

Example. Leroy Larson, a 16 year old boy, had an appendectomy. The outcome—"ambulates to bathroom unassisted within 48 hours"—would normally be realistic. However, because of an adverse reaction to his pain medication, Leroy was required to spend additional time in bed on IV fluids. Therefore, he was able to ambulate but required the assistance of the nurse. In this case, even though the outcome was not completely achieved, the client was progressing toward resolving the problem.

3. The client has not achieved the outcome and is not likely to in the future. At this point, the nurse should try to identify the reason why this is occurring. The first step is to reassess the problem or response to see if it was accurately identified. Next, new outcomes should be set. Perhaps the original outcome was unrealistic, given the resources of the client, nursing staff, or agency. Another possibility is that the client had no desire to achieve the outcome. Finally, the nursing interventions should be evaluated for their appropriateness in meeting the original outcome. Additional nursing approaches should be identified and initiated.

Example. Ellen Black is a 52 year old woman who has recently separated from her husband. They have been married 25 years. Ellen visited the crisis intervention center to obtain counseling for her depression. The psychiatric nurse practitioner recommended that she join a support group consisting of divorced and widowed women. An outcome was agreed upon—that Ellen would "report less depression after attending three sessions." However, Ellen's depression increased over the next two weeks, and she also verbalized that she would rather not live any longer. The psychiatric nurse practitioner changed the plan of care. It included a new outcome: "Ellen will voluntarily admit herself to a mental health unit."

Documentation

The nurse documents the evaluation of outcome achievement on the client's medical record. Precise terminology is used that clearly describes the client's status.

The use of *basket* terms, such as "good day," "tolerated procedure well," or "appetite poor," should be avoided. It is far more helpful to describe what the client said or did that led to the conclusions.

Example. Outcome: Free of episodes of chest pain throughout each shift. To evaluate this outcome, the nurse would (1) ask the client to report any episodes of chest pain, and (2) observe for indications of chest pain during any interactions with the client.

Documentation of this client's status would include a notation: "To Radiology for chest x-ray at 1:00. Complained of substernal chest pain radiating to left arm upon return to room at 1:45."

 9–1 TEST YOURSELF

MAKING JUDGMENTS ABOUT THE CLIENT'S PROGRESS

In the following situations, identify whether
1. The client *has* achieved the outcome
2. The client is *in the process* of achieving the outcome
3. The client *has not* achieved the outcome or is unlikely to in the future

Situation 1
Terry McNiff is being seen in the college infirmary for follow-up after an episode of pneumonia.
Nurse: "Terry, how are you doing on your goal to stop smoking?"
Terry: "I just can't handle that right now. Final exams are next week. Besides, I like to smoke."

Situation 2
Ethel Gore is a resident in a nursing home who has recently had the flu. As part of her recuperation, the nurse and client have agreed upon the following outcome: "Ambulates to the dining room for meals." The progress notes for 6/30/85 read "ambulated to the dining room for meals without assistance."

Situation 3
Ken Howard is being monitored in a hypertension clinic. Ken and the nurse have established a goal of a four lb weight loss monthly. One month later the nurse weighs Ken and determines that he has lost three lb.

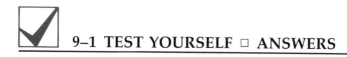

9–1 TEST YOURSELF □ ANSWERS

Situation 1
   The nurse-client interview indicates that Terry has not achieved the outcome, nor is he likely to in the future.

Situation 2
   Examination of the medical record reveals that Ethel has achieved the outcome.

Situation 3
   Direct observation indicates that Ken is in the process of achieving the outcome.

QUALITY ASSURANCE

Up to this point, the concept of evaluation has been discussed from the perspective of the individual nurse who evaluates the client's achievement of outcomes. The concept of *quality assurance* is defined as a planned and systematic evaluation of the care given to groups of clients. Quality assurance efforts began with a narrow focus. The client's chart was used as the sole measure of the quality of care. When this proved to be ineffective, the Joint Commission on Accreditation of Hospitals (JCAH) reconsidered its position. As a result, a variety of methods are now used to identify and eliminate factors that hinder effective care.

History

The concern for quality assurance is not new. Beginning in the 1600s, attention was paid to the rates of illness and death as indications of the state of health of the population.
   In 1916, Dr. Codman was one of the first to call upon hospitals to evaluate the quality of care delivered in their institutions. He said

> I am called eccentric for saying in public: that hospitals, if they wish to be sure of improvement, must find out what their results are. Must analyze their results to find their strong and weak points. Must compare their results with those of other hospitals. Must care for what cases they can care for well, and avoid attempting to care for cases which they are not qualified to care for well. Must assign the cases to members of the staff (for treatment) for better reasons than seniority, the calendar, or temporary convenience. Must welcome publicity not only for their successes, but for their errors, so that the public may give them their help when it is needed. Must promote members of the staff on a basis which gives due consideration to what they can and do accomplish for their patients. Such opinions will not be eccentric a few years hence. (Greeley, 1984.)

Although considered revolutionary in his day, Dr. Codman's points are valid and accepted today.

Shortly after World War I, the demand for critical evaluation of health care began to escalate. The pressures by consumers for some type of systematic evaluation culminated in the passage of legislation. In 1972, Congress mandated professional review of health care services, singling out the care delivered to clients on Medicare (people over 65 years of age), Medicaid (low income populations), and Maternal-Child Health programs. Professional Standards Review Organizations (PSROs) were created. In the 1980s the title of these organizations has become Professional Review Organizations (PROs), and their structure has been somewhat altered. The mission of the PSROs and the PROs is generally the same:

1. To ensure that all health care reimbursed from federal funds is necessary;

2. To ensure that care meets professional standards;

3. To require that care be provided economically in an appropriate setting.

The legislation described was based on the concept of peer review. This means that members of a profession that delivers a specific type of health care, such as medicine or nursing, should develop the bases for evaluation of that care. They should also complete the process of evaluation (Gordon, 1982).

During 1972, the JCAH revised its standards. It adopted the requirement that hospitals conduct systematic evaluations of the quality of care given to all clients (not just Medicare, Medicaid, and Maternal-Child Health clients).

Types of Evaluations

There are three different types of systematic evaluations or audits.

Structure

This type of evaluation focuses on the structure of care. It includes examination of the physical facilities, equipment, administration, policies, procedures, staffing, and qualifications of personnel. All of these factors influence the environment in which care is given. Figure 9–1 is an example of a structural audit that assesses the safety of the client's bedside environment.

Process

This form of evaluation encompasses the activities of the nurse as described by the nursing process. During the assessment phase, the nurse evaluates the data for completeness and accuracy and compares them with previous observations about the client. Together the nurse and client validate the nursing diagnosis. The evaluation component of the planning

MERCER MEDICAL CENTER

Nursing Department

CLIENT SAFETY CHECK

Instructions:

Review 10 clients on each unit   Date: _____

Review to be done by L.P.N.   Time: _____

Review odd number rooms, Bed B.   Unit: _____

SAFETY EVALUATION	YES	NO	EXPECTED COMPLIANCE
1. Identification bracelet in place?			100%
2. Name on bed?			100%
3. Call bell within reach?			100%
4. Bedside cabinet within reach?			100%
5. If applicable, telephone within reach?			100%
6. Drinking water within reach, if allowed?			100%
7. Is the light cord accessible?			100%
8. Bed in lowest position?			100%
9. Bed wheels in locked position?			100%
10. Bed crank recessed?			100%
11. If smoking allowed, proper receptacles?			100%
12. "No Smoking" sign in view, if O_2 in use?			100%
13. If patient is ambulatory with IV, IV pole on appropriate side of bed?			100%
14. Bed IV pole in center or bottom position on bed?			100%
15. If patient has foley:			
a. is it safely attached to leg?			100%
b. is it safely attached to bed?			100%
16. If restraints ordered, applied safely?			100%
17. Minimal bedside clutter?			100%
18. No medications found at bedside?			100%

NOTE: Report unsafe conditions to charge nurse.

Figure 9–1 □ Example of a structural audit. (Courtesy of Mercer Medical Center, Trenton, NJ.)

phase includes setting priorities among the identified nursing diagnoses and examining the outcomes and nursing orders for their potential usefulness. Evaluation in the implementation phase involves assessing the results of the nursing interventions. All of these activities constitute process evaluation. Figure 9–2 shows an example of a process evaluation of the nurse's medication administration skills.

MERCER MEDICAL CENTER MEDICATION SUPERVISION CHECKLIST FOR RN Name: _____ Date: _____	DATE	YES	NO	NOT OBSERVED	COMMENTS
GENERAL PROCEDURES					
1. Counts controlled drugs with oncoming and off-going shifts.					
2. Makes IV rounds to assess appropriate information (e.g., flow rate, site, type, and amount of solution).					
3. Notes information pertinent to accurate drug administration (e.g., NPO, x-ray, pre-op, I & O).					
*4. Checks medication Kardex for stat and single order medications and administers at ordered times.					
5. Checks transcription of medications with MD's order according to hospital policy.					
6. Checks Kardex for expired drugs according to hospital policy and takes appropriate action.					
7. Verbalizes hospital policy for medication error.					
8. Verbalizes hospital procedure for obtaining missing medication.					
*9. Properly documents omitted medication.					
10. Verbalizes hospital policy regarding syringe control.					
PREPARATION AND ADMINISTRATION					
1. Takes medication card to patient area.					
2. Prepares medication using following rules: a. Starts at top of medication Kardex and pours one medication at a time.					
*b. Checks label on drug against order in medication Kardex.					
*c. Accurately identifies the drug if a substitution by pharmacy has occurred.					
d. If not previously done, writes name of substitution medication under name of ordered medication on medication Kardex.					
*e. Pours correct dose.					

Figure 9–2 □ Example of a process evaluation. (Courtesy of Mercer Medical Center, Trenton, NJ.)

Illustration continued on following page.

MEDICATION SUPERVISION CHECKLIST FOR RN *Continued*	DATE	YES	NO	NOT OBSERVED	COMMENTS
f. Removes unit dose from the package only at patient bedside (if applicable).					
3. Administers medication using following rules: *a. Correctly identifies the patient by calling by name, asking the patient's name, and looking at ID bracelet.					
*b. Observes the patient swallowing pills.					
*c. Takes and records apical pulse when administering digitalis preparations and takes other vital signs as indicated.					
*4. For parenteral administration, chooses correct drug, dose, and time.					
5. Utilizes proper technique to draw up medication.					
6. Selects proper gauge and length of needle for patient.					
*7. Utilizes proper injection technique in site selection and administration.					
8. Destroys needle and/or syringe correctly.					
*9. Documents all medication administration in appropriate area on Kardex.					
10. Correctly records injection sites.					
*11. Identifies initials in signature column.					
*12. Records controlled drug administration properly.					
*13. When asked, can describe the action, side effects, and nursing implications of all medications administered. If unsure, seeks appropriate information.					
14. Administers intravenous fluids in accordance with hospital policy: *a. Maintains sterility of closed system.					
*b. Maintains IV fluid administration at ordered rates in conjunction with nurse assigned to patient.					
*c. Accurately labels IV solution according to rate of administration and medications added, if any.					

Figure 9–2 □ *Continued*

Illustration continued on opposite page.

MEDICATION SUPERVISION CHECKLIST FOR RN *Continued*	DATE	YES	NO	NOT OBSERVED	COMMENTS
*d. Checks site of patency and absence of inflammatory signs and symptoms and takes appropriate action.					
*15. Prepares IV medications using proper amount and type of diluent.					
*16. Administers IV medications at the correct rate.					
*17. Seeks appropriate information about incompatibilities when administering IV medications.					
*18. Administers blood and blood products according to hospital policy.					
19. When indicated, offers patient information about medications that he/she is receiving, i.e., name, action, and side effects.					
20. Documents patient education given about medications.					
21. Uses nursing judgment in questioning a dosage amount.					
*22. Uses nursing judgment in withholding a dose of medication.					
23. Asks questions when in doubt.					
24. Leaves medications cart clean and ready for use by next shift.					

Shift: _____ Time: _____

Supervised by: _____

Date: _____

Comments and/or suggestions:

_____

_____

_____

Signature of Employee: _____

Date: _____

*Denotes critical behaviors.

Figure 9–2 □ *Continued*

Outcome

Outcome evaluations comprise examination of those behaviors or states of the client that are the end result of nursing interventions. Outcomes represent the results of care. Figure 9–3 is an example of an outcome evaluation for a group of clients with the diagnosis of post-op lower extremity amputation.

OUTCOME AUDIT

Diagnosis: Post-op lower extremity amputation

Outcome Criteria at Time of Discharge	Actual Compliance	Expected % Compliance
No evidence of skin breakdown over bony prominences		100
No evidence of contractures or stump deformity		100
Change position and transfers from bed to chair		100
Verbalizes discharge instructions regarding care of stump		100
Identifies symptoms to be reported to MD		100
Verbalizes feelings regarding loss of leg		100

Figure 9–3 □ Example of an outcome evaluation.

Steps of the Audit

The structure, process, and outcome aspects of care may be evaluated by following certain steps, as outlined in Table 9–1. These steps provide an organized method for identifying and defining the component to be studied. Data are gathered and analyzed, the reasons for the problem are investigated, remedial action is taken, and a reaudit is undertaken after a period of time.

1. Selection of the topic is the first step. This may be a medical or nursing diagnosis, a procedure such as completion of a certain form, the care of a group of clients with similar nursing needs, and so on.

2. The next step is the identification of the specific standards of care to be evaluated. Standards of care are comprehensive guides defining the

TABLE 9–1 □ **STEPS OF THE AUDIT**

1. Selection of the topic
2. Identification of specific standards of care to be evaluated
3. Development of criteria for review
4. Definition of expected performance levels
5. Collection of data
6. Analysis of the information
7. Identification and implementation of solutions
8. Reaudit

ideal client outcomes resulting from nursing interventions or behaviors. Sources for standards of care include nursing textbooks and articles, the American Nurses' Association, and legal decisions on nursing care issues. See Table 9–2 for the standards of care for clients undergoing intravenous therapy.

3. Criteria are established from the standards of care. Criteria are the measurable characteristics describing the expected behavior of the client or the nurse. Figure 9–4 is an example of the criteria developed for the evaluation of one component of the standards of care for the client undergoing intravenous therapy.

4. Expected compliance or performance levels are developed next. A performance level represents the percentage of times that the auditor would expect the criterion to be met. For example, if an outcome criterion for a client is "identifies side effects of medications," the expected performance level might be 100 percent. This means 100 percent of the clients should be able to do this. Some expected performance levels might be expressed as zero percent. For example, the desired percentage of clients experiencing drug reactions would be zero.

5. Collection of data occurs next. This is accomplished by direct observation, interviews, or chart reviews.

Direct Observation. Direct observation is one of the most reliable methods of evaluating the structure and outcomes of evaluation care. Structural

TABLE 9–2 □ **STANDARDS OF INTRAVENOUS THERAPY**

1. Initiated by physician's order
2. Initiated by IV certified nurse
3. Inserted utilizing aseptic technique
4. Site inspected every eight hours
5. Flow rate maintained per physician's order
6. Tubing changed every 48 hours
7. Dressing changed every 48 hours
8. Solution changed every 24 hours

components—such as the physical facilities, client care, environment, staffing, written policies, and procedures—are readily evaluated. The client's progress is measured by comparing the actual outcomes with the desired outcomes of care.

Interviews. Questionnaires or interviews with the client may be used to elicit information about the process or outcome components of care. Clients may be asked such questions as

Process Questions	Outcome Questions
□ "Is your call light answered promptly?" □ "Do you feel well cared for?" □ "Are you being treated with courtesy?"	□ "What time do you take your water pill?" □ "How would you describe what is wrong with you?" □ Where do you plan to go to obtain your dressings after you go home?"

Chart Review. Chart review is an important mechanism for gathering data about large numbers of clients. Structure, process, or outcome components of care may be audited by chart review. Several parts of the chart—such as admission history and physicals, progress notes, care plans, intake and output records, and flowsheets—may be used for audit purposes.

Computers have proved to be useful in audits of the medical records. When charts are stored on a computer, it is possible to retrieve certain

---

Intravenous Therapy
Standard #6—Intravenous tubing is changed every 48 hours
Instructions:
   Completed by RN.
   Every client on intravenous therapy is to be reviewed.

Criteria	% Yes	% No	Expected % Compliance
IV tubing changed q 48 hours			100
Tubing labeled with:			100
Date			
Time of change			
Nurse's initials			
Change recorded on IV Kardex			100

Figure 9–4 □ Criteria for evaluating the standards of care of patients on IV therapy. (Courtesy of Hamilton Hospital, Trenton, NJ.)

data readily through the use of numerical codes. Computer searches reduce the amount of human time involved in an audit.

Concurrent Review. Concurrent evaluation occurs while the client is under the care of the agency. Both process components and some aspects of outcome components may be assessed. One of the advantages of concurrent review is the ability to use several methods of data gathering. Examples include observation of the performance of nursing care, interviews with the client, and chart review. An additional advantage is the opportunity to provide immediate feedback to the nursing staff. The observer has the chance to intervene, if required, to improve the variables being assessed.

Example. A concurrent evaluation is being performed to examine the care of clients receiving hyperalimentation. During the course of the audit, the observer notes that the dressing over a client's catheter site has not been changed for four days (despite the agency's policy for the dressing to be changed three times a week). The observer may be able to take action to correct this situation.

Example. An outcome audit is designed to examine bowel training for clients with a diagnosis of "alterations in bowel elimination: constipation related to immobility." The auditor finds that several clients are constipated in spite of the efforts of the staff. The auditor is able to suggest new nursing interventions that are more successful.

Gallant and McLane (1979) noted a disadvantage of concurrent reviews that evaluate the quality of care. Studies based on interviews with clients showed that relatively small numbers of clients indicated dissatisfaction with their care. The authors postulated that this may have been indicative of client's low expectations and fear of reprisals. It is important to establish an atmosphere of open communication and trust in which the client feels free to share concerns without fear of the consequences.

Retrospective Review. Retrospective review occurs after the client has been discharged from the agency's care. The process or outcomes may be evaluated by questionnaires, client interviews (telephone or face-to-face), or examination of the client's chart. Telephone interviews are reasonably inexpensive and may assist in the identification of unexpected problems. They may also be a valuable marketing strategy for a hospital that is trying to communicate a positive, caring image to the public. Face-to-face interviews provide another option, although certain logistical problems must be overcome. These include the amount of time involved and the setting of the interview—at the hospital or in the client's home.

The postcare questionnaire is another method of assessing the client's

outcomes and level of satisfaction with the care received. The questionnaire is economical to use and can be distributed in large numbers.
Frequently, however, small numbers of clients complete and return the
questionnaire, which may reduce its usefulness.

Chart review is the most commonly used retrospective data collection
method. It is useful in gathering process or outcome data. One of its
advantages is the fact that deficits in care may become noticeable when
large numbers of records are examined. Additionally, the records are
readily accessible for review.

The use of retrospective records for evaluation is based on the
assumption that the information documented reflects the actual care given
or the outcomes achieved. If the chart lacks these data, it could mean that
the nursing care was not performed or the desired effects not achieved.
Unfortunately, many types of information are often missing from a chart.
The question then arises—are gaps in the record due to a deficiency in
documentation or a deficiency in the nursing process? Since a retrospective
audit is performed after the client has left the care of the agency, it is
often impossible to answer this question.

6. The next step after data collection is the analysis of the information.
This involves an evaluation of any discrepancies between the collected
data and the criteria. Possible reasons for the differences are identified.

7. Next, possible solutions for correcting the discrepancies are derived. The solutions may include better definitions of outcomes, education
of nurses, changes in the process of delivering nursing care, and so on.

8. After implementing the solutions, a reaudit is performed. The
reaudit is used to evaluate the effectiveness of the solutions.

JCAH Reconsiders Outcome Audits

After considering the various types of evaluation methods for judging the
quality of care, the Joint Commission on Accreditation of Hospitals
selected the retrospective chart review. It required hospitals that were
applying for accreditation to perform a certain number of audits per year.
In response to the JCAH recommendations, hospitals begin to establish
mechanisms for the performance of retrospective outcome audits. However, a few years after the JCAH recommendations were enforced, critics
began to identify the limitations of this type of audit. They recognized
the difficulty in relying on the chart as the sole source of data, as previously
discussed. Additionally, they believed that important information that
process audits could provide was being missed. Finally, the critics felt

that hospitals were so caught up in the act of auditing, they failed to follow through to correct deficiencies that were identified.

Limitations of Outcome Audits

Since the JCAH method focused on client outcomes, the process of care was not evaluated until certain outcome criteria were not met. Since means of providing care are just as important as the ends or outcome of care, both need to be evaluated (Barba et al, 1978).

If clients are unable to achieve certain outcomes, it is necessary to evaluate both the structure and the process aspects of care. The evaluation should be aimed at identifying structural factors that are interfering with attainment of the outcomes and the nursing interventions (process) required to correct the situation.

Example. An audit reveals that a group of diabetic clients is unable to identify the relationship between insulin, diet, and activity. The question arises: are the diabetics unable to do so because they were not taught the content or because they are unable to remember the information? An evaluation of the process determines that this information was taught in a group class. A structure evaluation identifies the problem: the class was taught in a busy lounge. The diabetics were unable to absorb the information because of the distractions. One solution might be to move the class to another room in the future and subsequently to conduct a reaudit. Thus, structure, process, and outcome evaluations must be performed to gain a true assessment of the quality of care.

Finally, a third limitation of outcome audits relates to the nature of nursing. Much of nursing focuses on psychosocial problems, such as the adaptation to illness. This leads to significant measurement problems, since the results of such activities may not be readily apparent. Changes in behavior and level of understanding are difficult to measure (Hegyvary and Hussman, 1976). Therefore, a concentration on outcome audits would overlook one of the more important components of quality nursing care. Evaluation of the psychosocial realm is more readily assessed through process audits.

Lack of Follow-Up on Deficiencies

The JCAH requirements stated that a certain number of audits were to be completed each year. Many agencies used specific medical diagnoses. This resulted in a random search for problems to meet the quota of audits, and auditing became an end in itself. The goal of such review should not have been the accumulation of vast quantities of impressive documents but rather the education of the staff so that discrepancies would be corrected and the quality of care upgraded. In some settings, the audit was done because it had to be done. There were little motivation for the self-correction that such peer review could have provided. Additionally the JCAH, when conducting accreditation visits, tended to concentrate on the process of auditing rather than on the ultimate goal. The overriding concern seemed to be the format in which the audit was presented, with little indication of any interest in corrective activities (McClure, 1978). This further reinforced the seeming lack of importance of follow-up on deficiencies.

Quality Assurance in the 1980s

In 1980, recognizing the deficiencies of the retrospective chart review audit, JCAH developed a new approach to quality assurance. The essential components of this new program are

- ☐ Identification of important or potential problems or related concerns in the care of patients;
- ☐ Objective assessment of the cause and scope of problems or concerns, including the determination of priorities for both investigating and resolving them;
- ☐ Implementation, by appropriate individuals or through designated mechanisms, of decisions or actions that are designed to eliminate, insofar as possible, identified problems;
- ☐ Monitoring activities designed to ensure that the desired result has been achieved and sustained;
- ☐ Documentation that reasonably substantiates the effectiveness of the overall problem to enhance patient care and to assure sound clinical performance (Skillicorn, 1980).

During the early 1980s, JCAH developed and revised the quality assurance standards. The new standards eliminated the requirements for a specific number of studies to be performed annually. Rather, it emphasized the need for a problem-focused approach to the review of the quality and appropriateness of care. The focus shifted from a passive retrospective review system to a systematic active search for deficiencies in client care. Additionally, JCAH stressed that any type of audit was permitted—outcome, process, or structural, so long as it achieved the goal of identifying problems to be rectified.

Economic changes in the health care industry have reinforced the need for aggressive quality assurance monitoring and intervention. The most expensive care is often associated with complications necessitating prolonged intensive care, multiple surgeries, and costly tests and drugs. Changes in hospital reimbursement meant that in many cases these costs could no longer be passed on to the client. Therefore, all care that was excessive in cost warranted close scrutiny (Lang, 1984).

In 1984, further refinement of the JCAH standards resulted in the development of a systematic, planned, and ongoing monitoring program. Specific failures of care are being carefully monitored, and corrective and preventive actions are being swiftly taken. Problem areas that are closely monitored are

☐ Complaints from clients and families
☐ Reports of conflicts among professional staff members
☐ Unplanned returns to the operating room
☐ Unplanned transfers to other hospitals
☐ Unplanned admission to critical care units
☐ Cardiopulmonary arrests
☐ In-house emergencies
☐ Clients leaving against medical advice
☐ Cancelled surgeries, repeated x-rays, and laboratory tests
☐ Injuries, accidents, or incidents (Lang, 1984)

In addition to shifting the focus to ongoing monitoring, the new JCAH guidelines emphasize the need for hospital-wide quality assurance. Although many departments in hospitals were previously performing audits, rarely was an effort made to coordinate all of these activities. The audits often revealed that deficiencies resulted from breakdown in the systems for providing care. For example, a nurse might make a medication error because the pharmacy was late in filling the order or sent the wrong medication. Unless the various departments work together, resolution of hospital-wide problems frequently does not occur. The quality assurance effort must include nurses, physicians, administrators, technicians, laboratory staff—in short, representatives of every major department. Quality assurance committees have been established to bring everyone together and coordinate the detection and resolution of problems. They have become part of the effort to control costs, operate hospital efficiently, and provide quality care.

SUMMARY

Evaluation is an ongoing process used to judge each component of the nursing process. The term is used most commonly to describe decisions made about the effectiveness of nursing interventions. Evaluation of the quality of care given to groups of clients has evolved from the use of the nursing audit alone to the concept of quality assurance. In the future, aggressive efforts to provide for quality nursing care will affect both the client and the economic well-being of health care facilities.

References

Barba M, Bennett B and Shaw W: The evaluation of patient care through use of ANA's standards of nursing practice. Supervisor Nurse 42–54, January 1978.

Gallant B and McLane A: Outcome criteria: a process for validation at the unit level. Journal of Nursing Administration 14–21, January 1979.

Gordon M: Nursing Diagnosis: Process and Application. New York: McGraw-Hill, 1982.

Greeley Associates: Continuous Monitoring and Data Based Quality Assurance. Salem, Wis: Greeley Associates, 1984.

Griffith J and Christensen P: Nursing Process. St. Louis: CV Mosby, 1982.

Hegyvary S and Hussman R: Nursing professional review. Journal of Nursing Administration 12–16, November 1976.

Lang D: Prospective quality assurance. Quality Review Bulletin 143–145, May 1984.

McClure M: The long road to accountability. Nursing Outlook 47–50, January 1978.

Skillicorn S: Quality and Accountability: A New Era in American Hospitals. San Francisco: Editorial Consultants, Inc., 1980.

Bibliography

Bower F: The Process of Planning Nursing Care. 3rd ed. St. Louis: CV Mosby, 1982.

Carnevali D: Nursing Care Planning: Diagnosis and Management. 3rd ed. Philadelphia: JB Lippincott, 1983.

Edmunds L: A computer assisted quality assurance model. Journal of Nursing Administration 36–43, March 1983.

Graham N: Quality Assurance in Hospitals: Strategies for Assessment and Implementation. Rockville, Md: Aspen Systems Corporation, 1982.

Hanna K: Nursing audit at a community hospital. Nursing Outlook 24(1):33–37, January 1976.

Hover J and Zimmer M: Nursing quality assurance: the Wisconsin system. Nursing Outlook 242–248, April 1978.

Laros J: Developing outcome criteria from a conceptual model. Nursing Outlook 25(5):333–336, May 1977.

Mayers M, Norby R, and Watson A: Quality Assurance for Patient Care: Nursing Perspectives. New York: Appleton-Century-Crofts, 1977.

Phaneuf M: The Nursing Audit: Self Regulation in Nursing Practice. 2nd ed. New York: Appleton-Century-Crofts, 1976.

Walczak R: JCAH quality assurance requirements. Journal of Quality Assurance 10–11, Spring 1984.

Appendices

APPENDIX A □ **HEAD-TO-TOE ASSESSMENT CRITERIA**

General Appearance
□ *Observations*—age, race, nutritional status, general health status, development
□ *Color*—pink, pale, red, jaundiced, mottled, blanched, cyanosis
□ *Skin*—pigmentation, vascularity, temperature, texture, turgor, lesions (type, color, size, shape, distribution), bruises, bleeding, scars, edema

Vital Signs
□ Temperature
□ *Pulses*—apical, radial (others when appropriate)
□ Respirations
□ *Blood pressure*—supine, sitting, right and left arms
□ Height and weight

Head and Face
□ Size, contour, symmetry, color, pain, tenderness, lesions, edema
□ *Scalp*—color, texture, scales, lumps, lesions, inflammation
□ *Face*—movement, expression, pigmentation, acne, tics, tremors, scars

Eyes
□ *Acuity*—visual loss, glasses, contacts, prosthesis, diplopia, photophobia, color vision, pain, burning
□ *Eyelids*—color, ptosis, edema, styes, exophthalmos
□ *Extraocular movement*—position and alignment of eyes, strabismus, nystagmus
□ *Conjunctiva*—color, discharge, vascular changes
□ *Iris*—color, markings
□ *Sclera*—color, vascularity, jaundice
□ *Pupils*—size, shape, equality, reaction to light

Ears
□ *Acuity*—hearing loss, aid, pain, tinnitus, sensitivity to sound
□ *External ear*—lobe, auricle, canal
□ *Inner ear*—vertigo

Nose
□ Smell, nasal size, symmetry, flaring, sneezing, deformities
□ *Mucosa*—color, edema, exudate, bleeding, furuncles, pain, tenderness
□ Sinus tenderness, pain

Mouth and Throat
□ Odor, pain, ability to speak, bite, chew, swallow, taste
□ *Lips*—color, symmetry, hydration, lesions, crusting, fever blisters, cracking, swelling, numbness, drooling
□ *Gums*—color, edema, bleeding, retraction, pain
□ *Teeth*—number, missing, caries, caps, dentures, sensitivity to heat, cold
□ *Tongue*—symmetry, color, size, hydration, markings, protrusion, ulcers, burning, swelling, coating
□ *Throat*—gag reflex, soreness, cough, sputum, hemoptysis
□ *Voice*—hoarseness, loss, change in pitch

Neck
□ Symmetry, movement, range of motion, masses, scars, pain, stiffness
□ *Trachea*—deviation, scars
□ *Thyroid*—size, shape, symmetry, tenderness, enlargement, nodules, scars

☐ *Vessels* (carotid, jugular)—quality, strength and symmetry of pulsations, bruits, venous distention
☐ *Lymph nodes*—size, shape, mobility, tenderness, enlargement

Chest
☐ Size, shape, symmetry, deformities, pain, tenderness
☐ *Skin*—color, rashes, scars, hair distribution, turgor, temperature, edema, crepitation
☐ *Breasts*—contour, symmetry, color, size, shape, inflammation, scars, masses (location, size, shape, mobility, tenderness), pain, dimpling, swelling
☐ *Nipples*—color, discharge, ulceration, bleeding, inversion, pain
☐ *Axillae*—nodes, enlargement, tenderness, rash, inflammation

Lungs
☐ *Breathing patterns*—rate, regularity, depth, ease, normal or adventitious, fremitus, use of accessory muscles
☐ *Sounds*—normal, adventitious, intensity, pitch, quality, duration, equality, vocal resonance

Heart
☐ *Cardiac patterns*—rate, rhythm, intensity, regularity, skipped or extra beats, point of maximum impulse
☐ Right and left cardiac borders, implanted pacemaker

Abdomen
☐ Size, color, contour, symmetry, fat, muscle tone, turgor, hair distribution, scars, umbilicus, striae, fetus, rashes, distention, abnormal pulsations
☐ *Sounds*—absent, hypoactive, hyperactive, normal, bruit
☐ Liver border, gastric air bubble, splenic dullness, air fluid, muscle spasm, rigidity, masses, guarding, tenderness, pain, rebound, bladder distention

Kidney
☐ Urinary output (amount, color, odor, sediment), frequency, urgency, hesitancy, burning, pain, dribbling, incontinence, hematuria, nocturia, oliguria

Genitalia
☐ *Female*—labia majora, minora, urethral and vaginal orifices, discharge, swelling, ulceration, nodules, masses, tenderness, pain
☐ *Male*—penis: discharge, ulceration, pain; scrotum: color, size, nodules, swelling, ulcerations, tenderness; testes: size, shape, swelling, masses, absence

Rectum
☐ Pigmentation, hemorrhoids, excoriation, rashes, abscess, pilonidal cyst, masses, lesions, tenderness, pain, itching, burning

Extremities
☐ Size, shape, symmetry, range of motion, temperature, color, pigmentation, scars, hematoma, bruises, rash, ulceration, numbness, paresis, swelling, prosthesis, fracture
☐ *Joints*—symmetry, active and passive mobility, deformities, stiffness, fixation, masses, swelling, fluid, bogginess, crepitation, pain, tenderness
☐ *Muscles*—symmetry, size, shape, tone, weakness, cramps, spasms, rigidity, tremor
☐ *Vessels*—symmetry and strength of pulses, venous filling, varicosities, phlebitis

Back
☐ Scars, sacral edema, spinal abnormalities, kyphosis, scoliosis, tenderness, pain

APPENDIX B □ BODY SYSTEMS ASSESSMENT CRITERIA

General Appearance
□ *Observations*—age, sex, race, height, weight, nutritional status, development

Vital Signs
□ Temperature
□ Pulse (rate)
□ Respirations
□ *Blood pressure*—supine, sitting, right and left arms

Neurological System
□ Level of consciousness
□ *Skull*—size, contour, symmetry, color, pain, tenderness, lesions, edema
□ *Eyes*—acuity, visual loss, glasses, contacts, prosthesis, diplopia, photophobia, color vision, pain, burning, eyelid ptosis, edema, styes, exophathlmos, extraocular movement, position and alignment, strabismus, nystagmus, conjunctival color, discharge, vascular changes, corneal reflex, scleral color, vascularity, jaundice, pupil size, shape, equality, reaction to light
□ *Neck*—symmetry, movement, range of motion, masses, scars, pain, stiffness, lymph node size, shape, mobility, tenderness, enlargement
□ *Reflexes*—Deep tendon reflexes (DTRs), Babinski, posturing

Musculoskeletal System
□ *Activity level*—prescribed, actual, range of motion
□ *Extremities*—size, shape, symmetry, temperature, color, pigmentation, scars, hematoma, bruises, rash, ulceration, numbness, paresis, swelling, prosthesis, fracture
□ *Joints*—symmetry, active and passive mobility, deformities, stiffness, fixation, masses, swelling, fluid, bogginess, crepitation, pain, tenderness
□ *Muscles*—symmetry, size, shape, tone, weakness, cramps, spasms, rigidity, tremors
□ *Back*—scars, sacral edema, spinal abnormalities, kyphosis, scoliosis, tenderness, pain

Respiratory System
□ *Nose*—smell, nasal size, symmetry, flaring, sneezing, deformities, mucosal color, edema, exudate, bleeding, furuncles, pain, tenderness, sinus pain
□ *Chest*—size, shape, symmetry, deformities, pain, tenderness, expansion, crepitation, tactile fremitus
□ *Trachea*—deviation, scars
□ *Breathing patterns*—rate, regularity, depth, ease, use of accessory muscles, cyanosis, clubbing
□ *Sounds*—normal, adventitious, intensity, pitch, quality, duration, equality, vocal resonance

Cardiovascular System
□ *Cardiac patterns*—rate, rhythm, intensity, regularity, skipped or extra beats, point of maximum impulse, bruit, thrills, murmurs, rubs
□ Precordial movements, neck veins, right and left cardiac borders, pacemaker

Gastrointestinal System
□ *Mouth and throat*—odor, pain, ability to speak, bite, chew, swallow, taste, tongue size, shape, protrusion, symmetry, color, hydration, markings, ulcers, burning, swelling, coating, gum color, edema, bleeding, retraction, pain, number of

teeth, absence, caries, caps, dentures, sensitivity to heat, cold, gag reflex, throat soreness, cough, sputum, hemoptysis
- *Abdomen*—size, color, contour, symmetry, fat, muscle tone, turgor, hair distribution, scars, umbilicus, striae, rashes, distention, abnormal pulsations, sounds: absent, hypoactive, hyperactive; tenderness, rigidity, free fluid, liver border, air bubble, splenic dullness, air rebound, muscle spasm, masses, guarding, pain
- *Rectum*—pigmentation, hemorrhoids, excoriation, rashes, abscess, pilonidal cyst, masses, lesions, tenderness, pain, itching, burning

Renal System
- *Urinary patterns*—amount, color, timing, odor, sediment, frequency, urgency, hesitancy, burning, pain, dribbling, incontinence, hematuria, nocturia, oliguria, change in stream, enuresis, flank pain, polyuria, retention, stress incontinence, bladder distention

Reproductive System
- *Male*—penis: discharge, ulceration, pain, size, prepuce; scrotum: size, color, nodules, swelling, ulceration, tenderness, pain; testes: size, shape, swelling, masses, absence
- *Female*—labia majora, minora, urethral and vaginal orifices, discharge, swelling, ulcerations, nodules, masses, tenderness, pain, pruritus, Pap smear, menstrual flow, menopause
- *Breasts*—contour, symmetry, color, shape, size, inflammation, scars, masses: location, size, shape, mobility, tenderness, pain; dimpling, swelling, nipples: color, discharge, ulceration, bleeding, inversion, pain; axillae: nodes, enlargement, tenderness, rash, inflammation

Integumentary System
- *Color*—pink, pale, red, jaundice, mottled, blanched, cyanotic
- *Patterns*—pigmentation, vascularity, temperature, texture, turgor, lesions (type, color, size, shape, distribution), bruises, bleeding, scars, edema, dryness, ecchymoses, masses (size, shape, location, mobility, tenderness), odors, petechiae, pruritus, bruises, bleeding, scars, edema

APPENDIX C □ FUNCTIONAL HEALTH PATTERN ASSESSMENT CRITERIA

Health Perception–Health Management
□ Description of health (usual, current), preventive measures, previous hospitalizations and expectations of current hospitalization, description of illness (onset, cause), prior treatment (including compliance, anticipated self-care problems)

Nutritional-Metabolic
□ Usual daily food and fluid intake, appetite, food restrictions or preferences, food supplements, recent weight change, swallowing, chewing, feeding problems

Elimination
□ *Bowel*—usual time, frequency, color, consistency, assistive devices (laxatives, suppositories, enemas), constipation, diarrhea
□ *Bladder*—usual frequency, problems with frequency, urgency, burning, retention, incontinence, dribbling, dysuria, polyuria, assistive devices
□ *Skin*—condition, color, temperature, turgor, lesions, edema, pruritus

Activity-Exercise
□ Usual daily/weekly activities, occupation, leisure-exercise patterns, limitations in ambulation, bathing, dressing, toileting, dyspnea, fatigue

Sleep-Rest
□ *Usual sleep pattern*—bedtime, hours, sleep aids, problems falling asleep, staying asleep, feeling rested

Cognitive-Perceptual
□ *Sensory deficits*—hearing, sight, touch, problems with vertigo, heat or cold sensitivity, ability to read, write

Self-Perception
□ Major concerns, health goals, self-description, effects of illness on self-perception, factors contributing to illness, recovery, health maintenance

Role-Relationship
□ *Communication*—language, clear and relevant speech, expression, understanding
□ *Relationships*—living arrangements, support system, family life, complaints (parenting, relatives, abuse, marital problems)

Sexuality-Reproductive
□ Changes anticipated or experienced because of condition (fertility, libido, erection, pregnancy, contraception, menstruation)

Coping–Stress Tolerance
□ Decision-making (independent, assisted), major life changes (past, future, desired), stress management (eat, sleep, take medication, seek help), comfort/security needs

Value-Belief
□ Sources of strength, meaning, religion (importance, type, frequency of practice), recent changes in values, beliefs, needs during hospitalization

---

Adapted from Gordon M: Nursing Diagnosis: Process and Applications. New York: McGraw-Hill, 1982.

Physical Assessment
□ General appearance, weight, and height
□ Eyes, appearance, drainage, pupils, vision
□ Mouth, mucous membranes, teeth
□ Hearing, acuity, aids
□ Pulses, rate, rhythm, volume
□ Respirations, rate, quality, sounds
□ Blood pressure
□ Temperature
□ Skin color, temperature, turgor, lesions, edema, pruritus
□ Functional ability, dominant hand, use of arms, legs, hands, strength, grasp, range of motion, gait, use of aids, weight-bearing
□ Mental status, orientation, memory, affects, eye contact

APPENDIX D □ MARGARET LUNNEY'S NURSING DIAGNOSIS SYSTEM

Margaret Lunney, a nursing educator, has developed a simplified system of nursing diagnosis that can be used in many different settings. Her system is in use in many different settings—acute care facilities as well as community health centers.

Lunney's nursing diagnoses have two parts. The first part communicates the functional behaviors that can be improved through nursing assistance. These behaviors promote, maintain, or restore health. The second part identifies the etiology or the factors worked with to bring about improvement in the client's problems.

In this system, the behaviors are considered patterns or processes, so these words are not included in the diagnostic statement. For example, the National Conference System's term "sleep pattern disturbance" becomes "sleep/wake" in Lunney's system; "alterations in thought processes" beecomes "alteration in thought."

The terms for functional behaviors used in the first part of the diagnostic statement are

□ Activity/rest
□ Comfort
□ Communication
□ Coping
□ Elimination
□ Growth and development
□ Independence/dependence
□ Learning
□ Lifestyle
□ Management of health

□ Management of therapeutic regimen
□ Nutrition
□ Oxygenation
□ Parenting
□ Protection*
□ Relationships
□ Self-concept
□ Sexuality
□ Sleep/wake
□ Thought

Margaret Lunney uses only three modifiers, as opposed to the National Conference System, which uses a variety such as "ineffective," "impaired," "deficit," "dysfunction," and "acute." Lunney's modifiers are always placed in front of the first part of the nursing diagnosis. They are as follows.

Alteration in—means that there is a change in a functional behavior pattern from one that has previously promoted or maintained health to one that does not. In other words, there is a change from the usual optimum for the client.

For example, a client who is constipated may have an "alteration in elimination." A person experiencing pain has an "alteration in comfort."

Potential alteration in—means that the client is at risk for adverse change, or there is a possibility of a change from the usual optimum for the client.

For example, a client scheduled for surgery tomorrow may have a "potential alteration in coping." The surgical client who is a heavy smoker may have a "potential alteration in oxygenation."

Dysfunction in— means that the client's usual (as opposed to altered) behavior is one that does not help promote or restore health. For example, the person who abuses alcohol or drugs may have a "dysfunction in coping." The client with diabetes who does not follow the diet may have a "dysfunction in management of illness."

---

*The term *protection* is used to describe any threat, either internal or external, to the safety or well-being of the client. For example, a client at risk of falling would have a diagnosis of "potential alteration in protection related to weakness." A client at risk for infection would have a diagnosis of "potential alteration in protection related to infectious process."

A typical first part of the diagnosis would include

	activity
Alteration in	or
	comfort
	communication
Potential alteration in	or
	coping
	elimination
Dysfunction in	or
	management of health

Some examples include
   Alteration in nutrition
   Potential alteration in independence
   Dysfunction in parenting
   Alteration in communication
   Potential alteration in relationships
   Dysfunction in sexuality

The second part of the diagnostic statement describes factors that contribute to the unhealthful response. These are the intrapersonal, interpersonal, and nonpersonal factors that the nurse can work with to restore or maintain healthy functional behaviors. Interpersonal factors reflect changes or deficits in structure or function that involve interactions between the client and others. Nonpersonal factors are those that exist in the environment and influence the client's behavior responses. See Table D–1 for examples of each.

COMPARISON OF NATIONAL CONFERENCE SYSTEM AND MARGARET LUNNEY'S SYSTEM (see Table D–2)

National Conference System	Margaret Lunney
1. Impaired verbal communication related to language barrier (speaks only German)	1. Alteration in communication related to langauge barrier (speaks only German)
2. Potential for injury related to impaired perception (eye patch)	2. Potential alteration in protection related to impaired perception (eye patch)
3. Sexual dysfunction related to fear of rejection	3. Dysfunction in sexuality related to fear of rejection
4. Diversional activity deficit related to prolonged isolation	4. Alteration in coping related to prolonged isolation
5. Ineffective individual coping related to lack of support systems	5. Dysfunction in coping related to lack of support systems
6. Knowledge deficit (insulin injections) related to lack of prior exposure to the procedure	6. Alteration in management of therapeutic regimen related to knowledge deficit re: insulin injections
7. Potential impairment of skin integrity related to irritating stomal drainage	7. Potential alteration in protection related to irritating stomal drainage
8. Fear related to unknown etiology	8. Alteration in coping (fear) related to unknown etiology

While the list of functional behaviors is considered to be complete, the list of interpersonal, intrapersonal, and nonpersonal factors is not. These are only examples of factors. The factors should be as specific as possible to assist the nurse in planning nursing interventions.

For example, if a nursing diagnosis states "alteration in management of health related to knowledge deficit," the nurse does not know how to treat the problem. The nursing diagnosis would be more clearly stated as "alteration in management of health related to knowledge deficit re: breathing exercises."

TABLE D–1 □ PROPOSED NURSING DIAGNOSES

Human Response (Part One)		Contributing Factors (Part Two)
Alteration in—	*Related*	*Intrapersonal changes*
Potential alteration in—	*to*	Feelings of hopelessness, anger, loneliness, rejection
Dysfunction in—		Fear of pain, death, intrusion, rejection
Activity/rest		Perception of reality, hospitalization
Comfort		Anxiety
Communication		Infectious process
Coping		Hemorrhage
Elimination		Fluid and electrolyte imbalance
Growth and development		Lack of trust, differentiation
Independence/dependence		Change in body image
Learning		Change in role
Lifestyle		Sensory deprivation or overload
Management of health		Decreased self-esteem, cardiac output, hearing, mobility, hydration, levels of consciousness
Management of therapeutic regimen		Knowledge deficit of alternatives, contributing variables, illness, hospitalization
Nutrition		Open area of skin
Oxygenation		
Parenting		*Interpersonal Changes*
Protection		Rejection of different lifestyle
Relationships		Attachment
Self-concept		Separation
Sexuality		Lack of maternal/infant bonding, affection
Sleep-wake		Language barrier
Thought		Cultural barrier
		Lack of support system
		Absence of father image
		Isolation
		Nonpersonal Factors
		Excess noise or heat
		Lack of meaningful stimuli

Adapted from Lunney M: Nursing diagnoses: refining the system. American Journal of Nursing 457, March 1982.

TABLE D–2 □ DIAGNOSTIC TERMINOLOGY—LUNNEY VS. THE NATIONAL CONFERENCE SYSTEM

Modification I. Many terms used in Lunney's system are the same or only slightly changed from those accepted by the National Conference System. But such qualifying phrases as "alteration in," "impaired," and "ineffective" have been dropped. Although qualifying phrases would be included in the diagnostic statement for a specific client, they are not part of the diagnostic category. Also dropped from the diagnostic categories are such modifiers as references to who the client is ("family," "individual"), the body part/system ("bowel," "urinary"), and symptoms that would be in the data ("constipation," "diarrhea").

Lunney	National Conference
Comfort	Comfort, alteration in pain
Communication	Communication, impaired verbal
Coping	Anxiety
	Coping, ineffective individual
	Coping, ineffective family: compromised
	Coping, ineffective family: disabling
	Coping, family: potential for growth
	Social isolation
Elimination	Bowel elimination, alteration in: constipation
	Bowel elimination, alteration in: diarrhea
	Bowel elimination, alteration in: incontinence
	Urinary elimination, alteration in patterns
Nutrition	Nutrition, alteration in: less than body requirements
	Nutrition, alteration in: more than body requirements
	Nutrition, alteration in: potential for more than body requirements
Parenting	Parenting, alteration in: actual or potential
Self-concept	Self-concept, disturbance in: body image, self-esteem, role performance, personal identity
Sexuality	Sexual dysfunction
Sleep/wake	Sleep pattern disturbance
Thought	Thought processes, alteration in

Modification II. Some terms were developed to replace those used in the National Conference's accepted diagnostic categories to express behaviors more accurately.

Lunney	National Conference
Independence/dependence	Home maintenance management, impaired
	Mobility, impaired physical
	Self-care deficit (specify level): feeding, bathing/hygiene, dressing/grooming, toileting
Learning	Knowledge deficit (specify)
Nutrition	Fluid volume deficit, actual

Table continued on following page

TABLE D–2 □ DIAGNOSTIC TERMINOLOGY—LUNNEY VS. THE NATIONAL CONFERENCE SYSTEM *Continued*

Lunney	National Conference
Nutrition	Fluid volume deficit, potential
	Fluid volume, alteration in: excess
Oxygenation	Airway clearance, ineffective
	Breathing pattern, ineffective
	Cardiac output, alteration in: decreased
	Gas exchange, impaired
	Tissue perfusion, alteration in: cerebral, cardiopulmonary, renal, gastrointestinal, peripheral
Protection	Injury, potential for

Modification III. Some new diagnostic categories were added to express behaviors essential for health that were not identified in the National Conference System.

Growth and development
Lifestyle
Management of health
Management of therapeutic regimen
Relationships

Modification IV. Some of the National Conference's accepted diagnostic categories were not included. These are terms that do not represent health behaviors that nurses assist people in promoting, maintaining, or restoring; they are factors that affect these behaviors. When the nurse finds that any of these factors is present and affecting health, it can be included in the second part of the diagnostic statement (e.g., "alteration in protection related to open area of skin").

Diversional activity, deficit
Family processes, alteration in
Fear
Grieving, anticipatory
Grieving, dysfunctional
Noncompliance (specify)
Oral mucous membrane, alteration in
Powerlessness
Rape trauma syndrome
Sensory perceptual alteration: visual, auditory, kinesthetic, gustatory, tactile, and olfactory perceptions
Skin integrity, impairment of: actual
Skin integrity, impairment of: potential
Spiritual distress (distress of the human spirit)
Violence, potential for

APPENDIX E □ OMAHA CLASSIFICATION
SCHEME

Visiting nurses function more independently than do nurses in acute care settings. The primary service rendered in a home health agency is nursing (Daulton, 1979).

As previously mentioned, many visiting nurses have been dissatisfied with the National Conference System because the wording is not entirely appropriate for community nursing. Nurses have found that the diagnostic labels in the system are useful for labeling the acute physical needs of the client. However, wording that relates to the less immediate problems, such as chronic, social, or emotional ones, is not readily available (Cell et al, 1984).

Community health nurses need to use nursing diagnoses for the same reasons that nurses in other settings do: (1) to enhance communication, (2) to define nursing practice, and (3) to facilitate documentation of increasingly complex health care problems.

History

In 1977, the Division of Nursing of the Health Resources Administration (a government agency) assisted the Visiting Nurses of Omaha to develop an effective system for classifying and recording client problems requiring nursing intervention. The goal was to come up with a useful classification scheme that could be computerized.

The labels in the scheme were derived from the actual practice of the visiting nurses of Omaha. Three agencies located in Iowa, Delaware, and Dallas acted as test agencies to refine the wording. The system is now being used in many community nursing associations throughout the country.

Description

The classification scheme is an orderly list of health problems diagnosed by nurses in a community health setting. There are two parts to the classification scheme—the problem and the expected outcome. The first part of the scheme will be discussed here because of its focus on nursing diagnosis. It has four components.

1. Four major domains
2. Names of the problems identified in each domain
3. Modifiers of these problems
4. Signs or symptoms of these problems

Each specific item is assigned a numerical code for agencies that wish to computerize the scheme.

Four Major Domains

The four major domains represent broad areas of client problems that are addressed by the community health nurse.

1. *Environmental*—refers to the material resources and physical surroundings of the home, neighborhood, and broader community in which the client lives.

2. *Psychosocial*—refers to the patterns of behavior, communication, relationship, and development of the client. This domain often describes the inability of the individual or family to interact positively with persons inside or outside the family unit.

Adapted from Visiting Nurse Association of Omaha, Nebraska: A Classification Scheme for Client Problems in Community Health Nursing. Washington, DC: US Department of Commerce—National Technical Information Service, 1980.

3. *Physiological*—refers to the functional status of processes that maintain life.
4. *Health behaviors*—refers to activities that maintain or promote wellness, promote recovery, or maximize rehabilitation.

Problem Labels

Each domain has its own problem labels specific to that domain. For example, the environmental domain covers such areas as income, sanitation, and safety hazards, while the psychosocial domain covers isolation, grief, and anxiety.

Modifiers

Modifiers describe the problem. They may describe the degree to which the problem is present, such as actual or potential deficit or impairment. Actual problems are abbreviated AP. Potential problems are abbreviated PP. Modifiers also describe the location of the problem, as in "safety hazards (problem): residence (modifier)" or "safety hazards (problem): neighborhood (modifier)" or "abuse (problem): child (modifier)."

Signs or Symptoms

These are general statements that condense more specific information about the client. The signs or symptoms are listed below each problem. The word "other" appears at the bottom of each list of signs and symptoms, indicating that the nurse may add additional signs.

The diagnostic statement consists of the problem, modifier, and signs and symptoms. For example, a client with little money who is able to buy only the necessities and cannot pay medical bills not covered by insurance would be described as follows.

Modifier	*Problem*	*Modifier*
(Actual Problem—AP)	Income	Deficit

Signs	Low income
or	High medical expense not covered by insurance
Symptoms:	Able to buy only necessities

A client taking a medication that could cause diarrhea, such as an antibiotic, would be described as follows.

Modifier	*Problem*	*Modifier*
(Potential Problem—PP)	Bowel function	Impairment

Sign: Diarrhea

The classification scheme, without numerical codes, is shown in Table E–1.

Text continued on page 280

COMPARISON OF NATIONAL CONFERENCE SYSTEM WITH OMAHA CLASSIFICATION SCHEME (OCS)

National Conference System	OCS
1. Impaired verbal communication related to language barrier (speaks only German)	1. (AP) Communication with community resources: impairment (a) language barrier
2. Potential for injury related to impaired perception	2. (AP) Vision: impairment (a) inability to see small print
3. Sexual dysfunction related to fear of rejection	3. (AP) Human sexuality: impairment (a) relates difficulty expressing intimacy
4. Diversional activity, deficit related to prolonged isolation	4. (AP) Isolation: social (a) lacks contact with friends, family
5. Ineffective individual coping related to lack of support systems	5. (AP) Behavior pattern: impairment (a) demonstrates difficulty coping
6. Knowledge deficit (insulin injections) related to lack of exposure to procedure	6. (AP) Technical procedure: deficit (a) unable to demonstrate procedure accurately
7. Potential impairment of skin integrity related to irritating stomal drainage	7. (PP) Integument: impairment (a) drainage
8. Fear related to unknown etiology	8. Anxiety: (a)undefined fears

TABLE E–1 □ OMAHA CLASSIFICATION SCHEME

Environmental

Income: Deficit
Low/no income
High medical expenses not covered by insurance
Expresses/demonstrates difficulty in understanding money management
Able to buy only necessities
Difficulty in buying necessities (e.g., food, clothing)

Sanitation: Deficit
Soiled living area
Inadequate/improper food storage/disposal
Insects/rodents present
Foul odor
Inadequate water supply
Inadequate sewage disposal

Safety Hazards: Residence
Structurally unsound
Inadequate heat
Steep stairs
Obstructed exits/entries
Cluttered living space
Unsafe storage of dangerous objects/substances
Unsafe mats and throw rugs
Lacks needed safety devices

Table continued on following page

TABLE E–1 □ **OMAHA CLASSIFICATION SCHEME** *Continued*

Environmental

Lead base paint present
Unsafe gas/electrical appliances

Safety Hazards: Neighborhood
High crime rate
High pollution level (e.g., noise, air, waste)
Uncontrolled animals
High traffic area

Psychosocial

Communication with Community Resources: Impairment
Unfamiliar with procedures for obtaining services (e.g., education, health care,
transportation, food, day care, recreation, furniture, clothing, religion)
Difficulty in understanding roles of service providers
Unable to communicate concerns to service providers
Expressed dissatisfaction with services provided
Language barrier

Isolation: Social
Lacks contact with family/friends
Alone most of time
Uses health care providers for social contact
Minimal outside stimulation/leisure time activities

Behavior Pattern: Impairment
Demonstrates inappropriate suspicion
Demonstrates inappropriate manipulation
Exhibits compulsive behavior
Demonstrates passive-aggressive behavior

Role Change: Impairment
Reversal of traditional male/female roles
Reversal of dependent/independent roles
Assumes new role with loss of previous role
Assumes additional role(s)

Interpersonal Conflict
Expresses disillusionment with relationship
Lacks shared activities
Incongruent values/goals
Poor interpersonal communication
Expresses prolonged, unrelieved stress

Grief
Exhibits shock and disbelief
Exhibits denial
Exhibits anger
Exhibits bargaining
Family/individual in conflicting stages of grief process
Exhibits nonacceptance

TABLE E–1 □ **OMAHA CLASSIFICATION SCHEME** *Continued*

Psychosocial

Confusion
  Diminished attention span
  Disoriented to time/place/person
  Forgetful
  Inability to do simple calculations
  Inability to concentrate

Depression
  Downcast/sad/tearful
  Expresses feelings of hopelessness/worthlessness
  Loss of interest/involvement in activity
  Excessive inward focus
  Flat affect (e.g., monotone speech, limited body language)
  Expresses wish to die
  Attempts suicide
  Fails to meet personal needs

Anxiety
  Expresses feelings of apprehension
  Irritable
  Undefined fear(s)
  Much purposeless activity
  Inappropriate concern over minor things
  Tremors
  Narrow perceptual focus to scattering of attention

Sexuality: Impairment
  Fails to recognize consequences of sexual behavior
  Relates difficulty in expressing intimacy
  Sexual identity confusion

Parenting: Impairment
  Provides restrictive environment
  Handles child with difficulty
  Expresses dissatisfaction with parenting role
  Communicates inappropriately with child
  Uses excessive/inadequate/inconsistent control
  Conveys expectations incongruent with child's level of growth and
    development
  Lacks skills for caretaking (e.g., feeding, bathing, elimination)
  Lacks consistent routine for caretaking (e.g., feeding, bathing, sleeping)
  Inappropriate health care for minor injuries/accidents

Neglect: Child/Adult
  Primary caretaker inappropriately relinquishes responsibilities
  Fails to recognize psychosocial needs of child/adult
  Inadequate/delayed medical care
  Poor personal/environmental hygiene
  Child/adult left alone inappropriately
  Child/adult lacks necessary supervision
  Child/adult lacks appropriate stimulation/care

Table continued on following page

TABLE E–1 □ **OMAHA CLASSIFICATION SCHEME** *Continued*

Psychosocial

Abuse: Child/Adult
   Harsh discipline
   Welts/bruises observed/reported
   Injury with questionable explanation
   Verbal attacks
   Child/adult exhibits fearful behavior
   Physical violence
   Scapegoating
   Child/adult consistently receives negative messages
   Sexual violence

Growth and Developmental Lag
   Abnormal results of development screening tests (improvised/standardized)
   Slow gain in weight/height/head circumference in relation to growth curve
   Behavior inappropriate for age

Physiological

Hearing: Impairment
   Unable to hear normal speech tones
   Limited/abnormal response to sound
   Favors one ear for listening
   Abnormal results of hearing screening test (improvised/standardized)

Vision: Impairment
   Difficulty in seeing/inability to see small print/calibrations (e.g., syringe, thermometer)
   Difficulty in seeing/inability to see distant objects
   Difficulty in seeing/inability to see close objects
   Limited/abnormal response to visual stimuli
   Abnormal results of vision screening test (improvised/standardized)
   Squinting/blinking/tearing/blurring
   Color blindness

Speech and Language: Impairment
   Lacks ability to speak
   Demonstrates inability to understand
   Relies on nonverbal communication
   Uses inappropriate sentence structure
   Demonstrates poor enunciation or clarity
   Uses words inappropriately

Dentition: Impairment
   Missing/broken teeth
   Decayed teeth
   Sore gums
   Ill-fitting dentures

Respiration: Impairment
   Abnormal breath patterns (e.g., shortness of breath, dyspnea)
   Cough
   Cyanosis (with or without activity)
   Abnormal sputum

TABLE E–1 □ **OMAHA CLASSIFICATION SCHEME** *Continued*

Physiological

Noisy respirations
Rhinorrhea
Abnormal breath sounds

Circulation: Impairment
   Edema
   Cramping/pain of extremities
   Decreased pulses
   Discoloration of skin/cyanosis
   Temperature change in affected area
   Varicosities
   Syncopal episodes
   Abnormal blood pressure reading
   Pulse deficit
   Irregular heart rate
   Excessively rapid/slow heart rate
   Reports anginal pain
   Abnormal heart sounds

Neuromusculoskeletal Function: Impairment
   Limited range of motion (e.g., ROM/contractures)
   Poor coordination
   Gait/ambulation disturbance
   Decreased muscle strength/muscle tightness
   Inability to manage activities of daily living
   Tremors

Digestive Function: Impairment
   Nausea/vomiting
   Difficulty in chewing/swallowing
   Indigestion/heartburn
   Anorexia
   Anemia
   Abnormal weight loss

Reproductive Function: Family Planning
   Inappropriate/insufficient knowledge of family planning method(s)
   Inaccurate/inconsistent use of family planning method(s)
   Dissatisfied with present family planning method

Reproductive Function: Pregnancy
   Inability to cope with changing body
   Lifestyle incongruent with physiological changes
   Minor discomforts
   Fears delivery procedure
   Inability to cope with present body needs

Reproductive Function: Impairment
   Unusual/abnormal discharge
   Abnormal menstrual patterns
   Unusual changes in breasts
   Unusual changes in testicles/penis
   Dyspareunia (i.e., painful intercourse)

Table continued on following page

TABLE E–1 □ **OMAHA CLASSIFICATION SCHEME** *Continued*

Physiological

Bowel Function: Impairment
 Diarrhea
 Constipation
 Pain with defecation
 Minimal bowel sounds
 Blood in stools
 Abnormal color
 Reports cramping/abdominal discomfort
 Increased frequency of stools
 Incontinent of stools

Urinary Function: Impairment
 Incontinent of urine
 Urgency/frequency
 Burning/painful urination
 Inability to empty bladder
 Nocturia
 Polyuria
 Oliguria
 Hematuria

Integument: Impairment
 Lesion (e.g., wound, burn, incision)
 Rash
 Hypertrophy of nails
 Excessively oily
 Inflammation
 Drainage

Pain
 Statement of client
 Elevated pulse/respirations/blood pressure
 Movement compensation
 Restless behavior
 Facial grimaces
 Pallor/sweating

Consciousness: Impairment
 Lacks response to normal stimuli (e.g., touch, noise)

Health Behaviors

Nutrition: Impairment
 Weight 10 percent more/less than average
 Lacks/exceeds established standards for daily caloric intake
 Lacks/exceeds intake of one or more essential food groups/nutrients
 Lacks/exceeds appropriate fluid intake
 Improper feeding schedule for age
 Emaciated/obese

Sleep and Rest Patterns: Impairment
 Sleep/rest pattern interferes with family lifestyle
 Wakes frequently during night

TABLE E–1 □ **OMAHA CLASSIFICATION SCHEME** *Continued*

Health Behaviors

Somnambulism (i.e., walks in sleep)
Insomnia
Nightmares
Insufficient sleep/rest for age/physical condition

Physical Activity: Impairment
Sedentary lifestyle
Lacks regular exercise routine
Type/amount of exercise inappropriate for age/physical condition

Personal Hygiene: Deficit
Dirty clothing
Dirty skin
Body odor
Matted/unclean hair
Unclean teeth
Halitosis

Substance: Misuse
Abuses nonprescription drugs (e.g., medications, alcohol, nicotine)
Unable to perform normal routines
Reflex disturbances
Demonstrates change in behavior

Therapeutic Regime Noncompliance: Medical/Dental Supervision
Fails to obtain routine medical/dental evaluation
Fails to seek care for symptoms requiring medical/dental evaluation
Fails to return as requested to physician/dentist
Lacks consistent source of medical/dental care
Medical/dental supervision sought by client but prescribed regime appears
   inadequate to meet client needs

Therapeutic Regime Noncompliance: Prescribed Treatment Plan
Fails to perform treatment as ordered
Fails to obtain needed equipment

Therapeutic Regime Noncompliance: Prescribed Medications
Deviates from prescribed dosage
Lacks system for taking medication
Medication improperly stored
Fails to obtain refills appropriately
Fails to obtain immunizations

Therapeutic Regime Noncompliance: Prescribed Diet
Inability to integrate dietary prescription into balanced nutritional daily pattern
Does not adhere to diet as prescribed

Technical Procedure: Deficit
Unable to demonstrate/relate procedure accurately
Requires nursing skill
Unable to perform procedure without assistance
Unable to operate special equipment correctly

Issues Surrounding the Use of OCS

Some negative reactions to the OCS have occurred because of the claim that it is a forced choice, closed system. In other words, the nurse must choose from one of the problem labels and does not have the option to create a unique label. Such a closed system implies that the total domain of nursing practice is already known. A sufficient level of professional education can ensure that visiting nurses will retain the professional judgment necessary to use the system consistently without being rigid (Gebbie, 1984).

Proponents of the Omaha Classification Scheme would counter that it is not a closed system. The nurse may add additional signs or symptoms if the problem is not described by existing terminology. Additionally, the nurse may create a problem label if necessary. In that event, the nurse is encouraged to contact the Visiting Nurses of Omaha to discuss the need for a new label.

Community health nurses in agencies using the system report a number of benefits.

1. Charting is accomplished faster since the wording is already developed.

2. It is easier to determine whether data are significant or extraneous because the signs or symptoms provide a guideline for sorting and evaluating.

3. The specificity of the problem names and the signs or symptoms provides the basis for planning intervention measures (Visiting Nurses Association of Omaha, 1980).

4. The OCS specifically identifies and classifies problems of clients who are being cared for in the community setting.

5. The OCS is problem-oriented, and because it is not limited to the organizational structure of a specific visiting nurse service, it is appropriate for use by any agency (New Jersey State Department of Health, 1983).

6. The OCS forces nurses to think in terms of nursing diagnoses, gives them clearly stated goals, and makes it easy to evaluate care.

References

Cell P, Gordon J, and Peters D: Implementing a nursing diagnoses system through research: the New Jersey experience. Home Health Care Nurse 26–32, January–February 1984.

Daulton J: Nursing diagnoses in a community health setting. Nursing Clinics of North America 14(3):525–531, September 1979.

Gebbie K: Nursing diagnosis: what is it and why does it exist? Nursing Diagnoses, Topics in Clinical Nursing 1–9, January 1984.

New Jersey State Department of Health: Implementation of the Omaha Classification Scheme in New Jersey. Trenton: Home Health Agency Assembly of New Jersey, 1983.

Visiting Nurse Association of Omaha, Nebraska: A Classification Scheme for Client Problems in Community Health Nursing. Washington, DC: US Department of Commerce—National Technical Information Service, 1980.

APPENDIX F □ STANDARDIZED MODIFIED CARE PLANS

Burns in Children

Nursing Diagnosis	Outcomes	Nursing Plan
1. Impairment of skin integrity related to inflammation, potential infection	By discharge, child will have a healed or grafted burn.	1. Assess burned area for edema, redness, or discharge q shift. 2. Keep dressings dry and clean. If necessary use Pampers over area at mealtime. 3. Strict isolation.
2. Potential fluid volume deficit related to electrolyte imbalance.	1. Throughtout hospitalization, balanced intake and output. 2. Electrolytes within normal limits for client.	1. Strict monitoring of intake and output (I & O). 2. Specific gravity q shift until ____ day of hospitalization. 3. Assess electrolytes daily. Report abnormalities to MD. 4. Assess pulses and temperature of extremities q4h, first three days of hospitalization. 5. Vital signs (VS) q2h.
3. Alteration in nutrition: less than body requirements related to increased metabolic demands.	By discharge, will return to admission weight.	1. Daily weight at ____ A.M. 2. Encourage po fluids. Give children under 1 year _____ (formula). Encourage children over 1 year to take high-protein, high-caloric feedings. 3. Assess child's food likes and dislikes. 4. Involve child/parent in planning diet.
4. Potential for injury related to home hazards.	By discharge, family will verbalize burn prevention knowledge.	1. Obtain history of how burn occurred. 2. Explore with family ways to prevent recurrence, such as _____. 3. Give family "A Handbook of Child Safety." 4. Encourage family to describe preventive measures they will implement at home.

Continued on following page

BURNS IN CHILDREN *Continued*

Nursing Diagnosis	Outcomes	Nursing Plan
5. Alteration in comfort: pain related to inflammation.	Expresses comfort after receiving comfort measures within ____ minutes.	1. Assess for pain q2h. 2. Medicate with _____ prior to dressing changes. 3. Document effects of pain medication. 4. Change of position q ____h. 5. Provide diversionary activities (specify) ____.
6. Disturbance in self-concept: body image related to fear of rejection.	Throughout hospitalization, verbalizes feelings about change in appearance.	1. Encourage client to verbalize feelings. 2. Encourage client to look at burned area. 3. If appropriate, involve in dressing changes and skin care. 4. Assist in performing bedside exercises to increase self-care and enhance self-image.

CEREBROVASCULAR ACCIDENT

Nursing Diagnosis	Outcomes	Nursing Plan
1. Impaired physical mobility related to decreased function of L/R side.	1. Client and family demonstrate ability to perform range of motion exercises on affected side and to position correctly within ____ days. 2. Transfers from bed to wheelchair with assistance by time of discharge.	1. Maintain correct body alignment using assistive devices (specify): ____ Splints ____ Pillows ____ Sandbags ____ Footboard ____ Trochanter rolls ____ Foot drop protectors 2. Range of motion exercises at least tid or per physical therapy (specify) _____. 3. Instruct client and family in ☐ Range of motion activities ☐ Bed to chair transfer ☐ Position in bed (avoid high Fowler's position—leads to hip flexion)

CEREBROVASCULAR ACCIDENT *Continued*		
Nursing Diagnosis	**Outcomes**	**Nursing Plan**
2. Impaired verbal communication related to deficit of speech or comprehension.	1. Communicates needs effectively using communication aids. 2. Exhibits minimal frustration when communicating.	1. Diminish external distractions when communicating. 2. Use short, simple yes-and-no questions and gestures when communicating. 3. Speak slowly and allow adequate time for response. 4. Use all interactions to stimulate speech. 5. Use communication aid (specify) _____. 6. Obtain speech therapy consult (date: _____).
3. Alteration in urinary elimination patterns related to incontinence or retention.	1. Continent of urine. 2. Voids at least 250 ml q8h.	1. Monitor I & O. 2. Fluid intake of ____ml a day (specify). ____ 7–3 ____3–11 ____ 11–7 3. Limit po fluids after 8 P.M. 4. Maintain continence (check one) ____ Urosheath ____ Catheter ____ Bladder training (specify) _____ .
4. Alteration in bowel elimination: constipation related to diminished nutrition, immobility, and lack of response to defecation impulse.	BM without incontinence q ____day	1. If no BM for two days, initiate bowel regime (check which apply) ____ Check for impaction ____ Determine normal patterns ____ Obtain order for suppository qod ____ Stool softener daily ____ High fiber diet ____ Dietary consult (date: _____)
5. Self-care deficit: feeding, bathing, dressing related to diminished function L/R side.	By the time of discharge, demonstrates progress toward independence in personal hygiene, dressing, and ambulation.	1. Have client use unaffected hand to bathe and feed self.

Continued on following page

CEREBROVASCULAR ACCIDENT *Continued*

Nursing Diagnosis	Outcomes	Nursing Plan
		2. Obtain occupational therapy consult for training in self-care.
		3. For ambulation, use assistive device established by physical therapy.
		____ Knee splint
		____ Wheelchair
		____ Walker
		____ Quad cane
		4. Apply sling to affected arm. Instruct client or family to flex wrist q ____ h.
6. Alteration in nutrition: less than body requirements related to impaired swallowing.	1. Throughout hospitalization, no incidence of aspiration. 2. Swallows without choking. 3. By the time of discharge, feeds self with assistance.	1. Maintain suction set-up at bedside. 2. Provide for distraction-free, relaxed environment at mealtime. 3. Check for gag reflex prior to oral intake. 4. Sit upright during and one-half hour after meals. 5. Provide foods that can be eaten with one hand. 6. Place food within visual field. 7. Teach client to place foods on unaffected side of mouth. 8. Instruct client to flex neck and concentrate while swallowing. 9. Provide high texture foods. 10. Oral hygiene after every meal. 11. Weigh q ____ days.
7. Potential ineffective airway clearance related to immobility.	Exhibits no signs and symptoms of respiratory infection throughout hospitalization.	1. Change position q ____ h. 2. Encourage coughing or suction when indicated.

CEREBROVASCULAR ACCIDENT *Continued*

Nursing Diagnosis	Outcomes	Nursing Plan
		3. Provide mouth care pc and hs (specify) _____.
		4. Encourage breathing exercises (specify) ___.
8. Potential for injury related to visual changes, decreased sensation, confusion.	Experiences no injuries throughout hospitalization.	1. Keep frequently used objects on unaffected side.
		2. Approach from unaffected side.
		3. Teach client and family to safeguard areas of diminished sensation (e.g., heat/cold, pain, pressure).
		4. Use side rails.
		5. Restrain (specify) _____ _____.
9. Potential impairment of skin integrity related to diminished sensation, impaired mobility, and incontinence.	No evidence of skin breakdown throughout hospitalization.	1. Initiate turning schedule. Turn q ___ h (specify instructions) _____
		2. Use pressure-relieving devices (specify) _____. ___ Foam mattress ___ Heel and elbow protectors ___ Foot cradle
		3. Thoroughly wash and dry skin when incontinent.
		4. Massage pressure points with moisturizing agent q ___ h.
		5. Teach client and family to inspect skin areas frequently.
10. Alteration in thought process related to changes in emotional status.	Expresses feelings prior to discharge.	1. Encourage client to share feelings of depression, concerns re: changed body image.
		2. Explain to family that client may laugh or cry easily and inappropriately.

Continued on following page

Colostomy

Nursing Diagnosis	Outcomes	Nursing Plan
1. Potential alteration in bowel elimination related to obstruction.	1. Nasogastric (NG) tube drainage within normal limits (WNL) q8h. 2. Passage of flatus/discharge from the stoma by ____ post-op day. 3. By time of discharge, return of bowel function through the stoma.	1. Check NG tube patency. Irrigate with normal saline solution (NSS) q ____ h and prn. 2. Monitor NG tube contents. Chart color, amount of drainage q ____ h. 3. Observe for passage of flatus/drainage through stoma. 4. Notify MD if ostomy site is not functioning within ____ hours. 5. Check bowel sounds q shift. 6. Monitor for changes in stool consistency as nutritional intake progresses.
2. Potential for injury related to ☐ Decreased perfusion to stoma ☐ Contamination of wound by ostomy drainage.	1. Throughout hospitalization, pink- → red-colored stoma. 2. Demonstrates wound healing by time of discharge.	1. Monitor stoma q ____ h. Chart color, condition, and any discharge. 2. Notify MD immediately if stoma color is dusky or blackened. 3. Contain stomal drainage with appliance. Keep dressing over surgical site when changing ostomy appliance or emptying drainage. 4. Inspect incision q ____ h and document findings.
3. Potential impairment of skin integrity related to irritating stomal drainage.	During post-op period: 1. Peristomal skin free from excoriation 2. Stomal drainage contained by ostomy appliance.	1. Apply ostomy pouch immediately post-op (specify type) ____. *(Use skin barrier.)* 2. Change appliance q ____ days and prn. 3. Document condition of peristomal skin. 4. Clean stoma gently but thoroughly with ____.

COLOSTOMY *Continued*

Nursing Diagnosis	Outcomes	Nursing Plan
		5. Consult with stomal therapist (date: _____).
4. Potential alteration in comfort: pain related to ☐ Effects of surgery ☐ NG tube placement	1. Reports pain immediately. 2. Expresses comfort within ____ after initiation of comfort measures. 3. No evidence of pressure on nares.	1. Encourage client to report pain immediately. 2. Assess type, duration, and intensity of pain. 3. Administer medication per MD order. 4. Assess and document medication effects. 5. Apply skin prep to nares. Secure tube with tape, change daily and prn. 6. Mouth care (specify) ☐ Moisten lips with _____. ☐ Refresh mouth with _____. ☐ Provide cold water for rinsing but not swallowing.
5. Disturbance in self-concept related to change in body image.	1. Verbalizes feelings about ostomy to person of choice. 2. Expresses positive feelings about self daily. 3. Within ____ days post-op, views stoma.	1. Assist client to maintain own personal hygiene, bedclothes, apply make-up (specify) _____. 2. Spend at least ____ min per shift in room. 3. Encourage client/partner to ☐ Express feelings re: ostomy; ☐ View stoma. 4. Use open-ended questions. 5. Acknowledge feelings of anger/depression as normal. 6. Arrange for visitor with ostomy to provide realistic support (date: _____).
6. Sexual dysfunction related to ☐ Feelings of rejection ☐ Effects of surgery	By the time of discharge, client/partner will verbalize concerns.	1. Offer realistic information to prevent misconceptions.

Continued on following page

COLOSTOMY *Continued*

Nursing Diagnosis	Outcomes	Nursing Plan
		2. Create opportunity for verbalization of fears (specify) _____.
		3. Encourage client/partner to seek professional guidance if a problem develops.
7. Knowledge deficit related to care of ostomy.	By time of discharge: 1. Client or family member will be able to demonstrate care of the ostomy appliance; 2. Client/family will be able to describe dietary management for proper regulation of ostomy upon discharge.	1. Assess for readiness to learn ostomy care. 2. Initiate teaching plan and provide teaching packet (date: _____). 3. Give step-by-step explanation to client. 4. Include family member(s) in teaching. 5. Provide list of ostomy equipment and suggested places of purchase. 6. Social Service referral for follow-up (date: _____). 7. Review prescribed diet. Dietary consult if necessary. 8. If no specific diet order, review foods to avoid for gas, odor formation, and blockage.

HYPEREMESIS GRAVIDARUM (PATHOLOGICAL VOMITING IN PREGNANCY)

Nursing Diagnosis	Outcomes	Nursing Plan
1. Alteration in nutrition (less than body requirements) related to dehydration.	Throughout hospitalization: 1. No weight loss; 2. Decreased vomiting; 3. Able to tolerate diet; 4. Electrolytes within normal limits; 5. Free of signs of dehydration—coated tongue, dry mucous membranes, dry skin.	1. Daily weight at ____ A.M. 2. NPO initially for ____ h. 3. Provide vitamins and IV calories to maintain nutrition as ordered. 4. Consult dietician. 5. Reinforce need for calorie counting and eating snacks.

HYPEREMESIS GRAVIDARUM (PATHOLOGICAL VOMITING IN PREGNANCY) *Continued*

Nursing Diagnosis	Outcomes	Nursing Plan
		6. Check urine for ketones and proteins every voiding and while receiving IVs, then q shift when tolerating diet. 7. Check urine specific gravity q ___ h. 8. Monitor I & O. 9. Assess lab work and notify MD if outside normal range.
2. Potential ineffective individual coping related to psychological adjustment to pregnancy and role change.	Throughout hospitalization, verbalizes feelings about pregnancy.	1. Encourage client to verbalize feelings about pregnancy and history of conception. 2. To enable the client to visualize fetus, show pictures of developing fetus. 3. Encourage rest by providing quiet environment. 4. Suggest limitation of visitors.
3. Knowledge deficit related to diet, activity, and physiological changes of pregnancy.	Prior to discharge, verbalizes understanding of diet, activity, and physiological changes of pregnancy.	1. Give client booklets on diet and exercise. 2. Explain physiological changes of each trimester. 3. Explain need for rest and healthy sleep patterns when discharged.

PNEUMONIA

Nursing Diagnosis	Outcomes	Nursing Plan
1. Impaired gas exchange related to retained secretions.	1. Resumes normal breathing patterns within ___. 2. Lung sounds clear bilaterally. 3. Chest x-ray clear by time of discharge. 4. Within 48 h temp ↓ to ___°.	1. Maintain bedrest for ___h. 2. Change position q ___ h to facilitate lung expansion. 3. Monitor for change in respiratory status q ___ h.

Continued on following page

PNEUMONIA *Continued*		
Nursing Diagnosis	**Outcomes**	**Nursing Plan**
		4. Auscultate lung sounds q ___ h.
		5. Coughing and deep breathing exercises q ___ h.
		6. Intermittent positive-pressure breathing (IPPB) q ___ (specify).
		7. Chest physical therapy (PT) and postural drainage q ___ h (specify) ___.
		8. O₂ at ___ l/min via ___ Nasal cannula ___ Mask
		9. Assess for alteration in level of consciousness q ___ h. Document restlessness, confusion, agitation.
		10. Monitor arterial blood gases (ABG) results as ordered.
		11. If unable to cough productively, suction q ___ h and prn using aseptic technique (specify). ___ Oropharyngeal suction ___ Nasotracheal suction ___ Endotracheal suction Give mouth care after suctioning.
		12. Note amount, consistency, color, and odor of secretions.
		13. Collect sputum cultures as ordered (culture sent: ___).
		14. Monitor culture results—notify physician.
		15. Monitor chest x-ray reports.
		16. Monitor vital signs q ___ h. (Rectal temps if indicated.)

Pneumonia *Continued*		
Nursing Diagnosis	**Outcomes**	**Nursing Plan**
		17. Administer antibiotics/antipyretics as ordered to decrease O_2 consumption.
		18. Take measures to reduce body temperature.
		□ Utilize hypothermia blanket for temp ↑ ____ °.
		□ Give tepid or alcohol sponge baths for temp ↑ ____ °.
2. Potential for fluid volume deficit related to decreased oral intake.	Within 24 hours 1. Balanced I & O; 2. Electrolytes WNL.	1. Accurate I & O q shift. 2. Maintain IV per MD order. 3. Force fluids if indicated (specify) ____ ml daily. ____ 7–3 ____ 3–11 ____ 11–7 4. Assess skin turgor. 5. Monitor electrolyte results.
3. Alteration in comfort realted to □ Coughing episodes □ Dry mucous membranes	1. Rest periods will not be interrupted by coughing. 2. Moist mucous membranes.	1. Assist during coughing episodes. □ Sit upright. □ Splint chest with pillows. 2. Institute measures to decrease frequency of coughing. □ Mouth care prn. □ Sips of water. □ Hard candy if it helps control coughing. □ Maintain planned rest periods. □ Discourage talking. □ Limit visitors. □ Keep environment free from flowers, smoke, and dust.
4. Alteration in nutrition (less than body requirements) related to anorexia.	1. No evidence of significant weight change.	1. Provide small frequent meals. 2. Assess likes/dislikes. 3. Encourage food from home if permitted.

Continued on following page

	PNEUMONIA *Continued*	
Nursing Diagnosis	**Outcomes**	**Nursing Plan**
		4. Obtain dietary consult (date: _____).
		5. Monitor food intake.
		6. Supplemental feeding prn (specify) _____.
		7. Weight daily at ____ .
5. Knowledge deficit related to ☐ Risk factors ☐ Medications.	By time of discharge: 1. Identifies risk factors; 2. Verbalizes ways to prevent disease recurrence;	1. Instruct client or family to ☐ Limit exercise and activity to tolerance; ☐ Plan rest periods during the day; ☐ Perform coughing and deep breathing exercises qid for 6–8 weeks; ☐ Keep warm—avoid chilling and persons with infections, especially upper respiratory infection (URI). 2. Report following symptoms to physician: ☐ Increased temp; ☐ Diaphoresis; ☐ Difficult breathing; ☐ Persistent cough; ☐ Cold or flu.
	3. States names of medications, dosage, time of administration, action, and major side effects.	3. Review medication schedule and provide client with information. 4. Instruct client to avoid taking over-the-counter drugs without first checking with physician.

	THORACOTOMY	
Nursing Diagnosis	**Outcomes**	**Nursing Plan**
1. Impaired gas exchange related to ☐ Retained secretions; ☐ Hypoventilation.	Within 48 hours: 1. No evidence of respiratory distress; 2. Breath sounds present bilaterally; 3. ABG WNL for client.	1. Administer humidified O_2 at ____ liters/minute to enhance oxygenation.

THORACOTOMY *Continued*		
Nursing Diagnosis	**Outcomes**	**Nursing Plan**
		2. Monitor respirations q ___ h. Note dyspnea, tachypnea, stridor.
		3. Auscultate lungs—note depth and pattern.
		4. Assess for restlessness.
		5. Monitor ABG.
		6. Encourage coughing and deep breathing q ___ .
		7. Suction if unable to expectorate.

2. Potential for injury related to
☐ Clotting in chest tube
☐ Tubing disconnection
	While chest tube in place:
	1. Free flow of blood/air from pleural cavity;
	2. Intact drainage system;
		1. Maintain patent drainage system: milk chest tubes q ___ min × ___ then q ___ h.
		2. Monitor fluid levels in drainage system q ___ . Fill prn.
		  ☐ Avoid kinking tubing.
		  ☐ Tape all tubing connections.
		  ☐ Clamps at bedside.
		  ☐ Do not raise drainage system above level of chest.

☐ Air leak	3. No evidence of air leak.	3. Observe for indications of air leak.
		  ☐ Air bubbling down tubing.
		  ☐ Signs and symptoms of pneumothorax, shortness of breath (SOB), dyspnea, tachypnea.
		4. Monitor chest drainage q1h and report if > 100 ml/h. Check dressing for unusual bleeding.

3. Alteration in comfort: pain related to effects of surgery.	1. Reports pain immediately. 2. Expresses comfort within 1 h after initiation of comfort measures.	1. Explain pain regime to client/family (specify) _____. 2. Assess for location, intensity q ___ h.

Continued on following page

THORACOTOMY *Continued*		
Nursing Diagnosis	**Outcomes**	**Nursing Plan**
		3. Administer pain medication per MD order.
		4. Assess and document effects.
		5. Instruct client to avoid lying on chest tube site.
4. Impaired physical mobility related to pain, fear of movement.	By time of discharge, full ROM of ___ arm.	1. Explain need for turning and arm movement.
		2. ROM to ___ arm and shoulder q ___.
		3. Obtain consult with physical therapy (date: _____).
5. Knowledge deficit related to postdischarge care.	Prior to discharge: 1. Demonstrates wound care; 2. States symptoms to report to MD; 3. Verbalizes activity limitations.	1. Instruct client to □ Perform wound care; □ Report redness, swelling and increased temp, incisional drainage; □ Report sudden pain, dyspnea, shortness of breath, bleeding, etc.; □ Avoid lifting activities until cleared by MD; □ Continue coughing and deep breathing; □ Schedule alternate periods of activity/rest; □ Avoid exposure to smoke, air pollution.

Index